Recent Advances in Male Reproductive System

Edited by Wei Wu

Published in London, United Kingdom

Recent Advances in Male Reproductive System
http://dx.doi.org/10.5772/intechopen.1000558
Edited by Wei Wu

Contributors
Gbolahan Oladele Obajimi, Bamgboye Morakinyo Afolabi, Yan Yuan, Peihao Wu, Yixuan Yan, Jing Wang, Jialin Feng, Jinqi Ma, Qiuqin Tang, Wei Wu, Yasuko Fujisawa, Ogata Tsutomu, Ahmed Atwa, Serag Eldin I. Elbehairi, Sayed Bakry, Ahmed B.M. Mehany, Mahmoud Ashry, Hussam Askar, Mohammad Y. Alfaifi, Murid Javed, Seang L. Tan, Ralf Herwig, Neelesh Kumar Maurya

First published in London, United Kingdom, 2023 by IntechOpen
IntechOpen is the global imprint of INTECHOPEN LIMITED, registered in England and Wales, registration number: 11086078, 5 Princes Gate Court, London, SW7 2QJ, United Kingdom

British Library Cataloguing-in-Publication Data
A catalogue record for this book is available from the British Library

Additional hard and PDF copies can be obtained from orders@intechopen.com

Recent Advances in Male Reproductive System
Edited by Wei Wu
p. cm.
Print ISBN 978-1-83769-736-6
Online ISBN 978-1-83769-735-9
eBook (PDF) ISBN 978-1-83769-737-3

Meet the editor

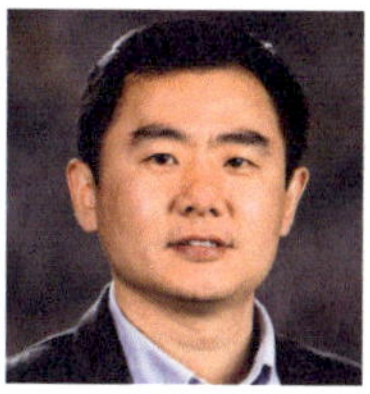

Dr. Wei Wu is a Professor and Associate Department Chair of the Department of Toxicology, Nanjing Medical University, China, where he received his Ph.D. in Toxicology. He was a guest researcher at the National Institute of Environmental Health Sciences (NIEHS) between 2017 and 2018. Dr. Wu is a member of different national and international societies in the fields of human reproduction and toxicology and has received awards from many national societies for the originality and quality of his projects. Dr. Wu has authored eighty-four peer-reviewed papers in international journals, edited five books, and collaborated on ten others. He has nineteen patents to his credit. He has organized four international conferences. Dr. Wu is also a reviewer for 108 journals.

Contents

Preface

Male factor infertility is responsible for about half of all cases of infertility, and thus, a sound understanding of its etiology and treatment options is important for the successful management of involuntary childlessness. Male factor infertility may result from several factors, including idiopathic, endocrine, environmental, anatomic, behavioral/lifestyle, and iatrogenic factors. Impaired male reproductive health has been linked to a decreased general health status, and severe male infertility has been associated with a higher risk of malignancy. This book discusses the physiological structure, function, common diseases and their risk factors, and treatments of the male reproductive system. We hope this book will not only meet the needs of professionals but also help the general reader. It provides a better understanding of how the male reproductive system operates and how to maintain and improve its health.

Chapter 1 discusses the epidemiology, etiology, evaluation, and management of male infertility.

Chapter 2 outlines the concept and phenotype of intergenerational and transgenerational inheritance induced by endocrine-disrupting chemicals, summarizes the recent achievements of important epigenetic molecular mechanisms, and provides a relevant theoretical basis for the protection of male fertility.

Chapter 3 discusses how intrauterine hyponutrition leads to male reproductive dysfunction and the contribution of epigenomic modifications in the development of testicular dysgenesis syndrome.

Chapter 4 focuses on refractory infertility diseases and their characteristics, as well as potential treatment strategies using stem cells as an alternative to assisted reproductive technology.

Chapter 5 discusses the advances in male infertility treatment through assisted reproductive technology.

Chapter 6 discusses the pathophysiology, physical principles, clinical presentation, and diagnosis of erectile dysfunction caused by cavernous leakage.

Chapter 7 overviews factors that influence libido and talks about how functional foods such as spinach, dark chocolate, peppers, green tea, oysters, crab, and pumpkin seeds, which contain neurotransmitters, affect libido.

There are many individuals who made this book a reality. The completion of this book would not have been possible without the efforts of numerous contributors.

I would like to thank Ms. Mirna Papuga at IntechOpen for her strong support from the inception to the completion of this book. I would also like to acknowledge my coauthors for their efforts.

Wei Wu
Department of Toxicology,
School of Public Health,
Nanjing Medical University,
Nanjing, China

Chapter 1

Male Infertility: Aetiology and Management in Contemporary Practice

Gbolahan Oladele Obajimi and Bamgboye Morakinyo Afolabi

Abstract

Human reproduction, a pas de deux, is dependent on the functional competence of both male and female reproductive systems. Male factor infertility accounts for about half of the causes of infertility and strictly affects about 7% of all men. While most cases are idiopathic, a smaller proportion can be adduced to a wide variety of causes generally classified as pre-testicular, testicular, and post-testicular. Extrinsic factors bordering on behaviour and habits which are generally modifiable, should be given due attention in the evaluation and initial management of male infertility. A range of investigations can be employed in the evaluation of male infertility, however, semen analysis, the least invasive and most cost effective, is prognostic but does not always guarantee fecundity as multiple interrelated factors have been implicated in male infertility. Treatment options though varied, aim at improving semen quality and assisted reproductive technique (ART) is offered in cases of severe male infertility. This chapter provides an overview of male factor infertility with a focus on investigation and contemporary management in a dynamic world. It further provides insights into advances in stem cell therapeutics and artificial intelligence.

Keywords: male infertility, aetiology, management, challenges, contemporary practice

1. Introduction

Infertility refers to the inability of a couple to achieve conception after one year of regular unprotected sexual intercourse [1]. Reproduction on the other hand is important for the continued existence of the human species as a means of compensation for death or disease. Involuntary childlessness is a pervasive medical condition that has been found to adversely affect the psychosocial wellbeing of the affected couple [2]. Infertility has been associated with an increased economic burden on both patient and the healthcare institution [3] and this burden is exaggerated in many low-income countries where funding through health insurance is lacking, and this further worsens the outlook for the infertile couple [4].

Infertility is estimated to globally affect about 8–12% of couples with both parties contributing equally to its incidence [5]. In the United Kingdom, it has been estimated that one in seven couples experience challenges with conception with the male partner contributing up to half of the cases [6], however, male infertility is thought to

 IntechOpen

strictly affect 7% of all men [7]. Impaired male reproductive health has been linked to a decreased general health status and severe male infertility has been associated with a higher risk of malignancy [8, 9].

Male factor infertility may result from several factors which include idiopathic, endocrine, environmental, anatomic, behavioural/lifestyle and iatrogenic factors. Idiopathic or unknown factors are the most prevalent and account for over half of the cases seen. Understanding the aetiology of male infertility is made easier by classifying them into pre-testicular, testicular, and post-testicular causes.

2. Epidemiology

A variety of health conditions can adversely affect male fertility and male reproductive disorders can be identified in about half of male partners of an infertile union. Male factor infertility evidenced by abnormal semen parameters is noted to affect about 7% of all men and its extreme form, azoospermia is found in 1% of the general population and in about 20% of patients attending a fertility clinic [10]. Evidence suggests that the health status of a male partner at the time of conception may affect the metabolic health and reproductive potential of the progeny [11].

Globally over the past five decades, sperm count has been reported to decline and a systematic review by Levine et al demonstrated a decline of between 50–60% between 1973 and 2011, further underscoring the rising contribution of male factor infertility [12]. Prognostic factors influencing the outcome of fertility management includes the duration of infertility, age of the female partner, disorders of semen production and the type of infertility which may be either primary or secondary. Despite advances in male reproductive health, progress in the management of male factor infertility has been limited and often restricted to assisted reproduction. Early diagnosis through prompt and thorough evaluation of the male reproductive system is critical in the successful management of male infertility. This chapter provides an overview of the aetiology and contemporary management strategies for male factor infertility especially in the context of advances in assisted reproductive technique.

3. Aetiology

The aetiology of male factor infertility has traditionally been classified as pre-testicular, testicular, and post-testicular factors and these factors have been viewed as congenital, acquired, or idiopathic. Idiopathic factors account for at least 50% of the causative factors of male infertility and a precise diagnosis is often lacking.

Congenital causes of male infertility include cryptorchidism (undescended testis), congenital absence of the vas deferens (CAVD), anorchia, genetic endocrinopathy, genetic abnormalities and Robertsonian translocations. Acquired factors on the other hand range from infectious morbidities to trauma. These include recurrent urogenital infections leading to urogenital tract obstructions, inflammatory conditions such as epididymitis and orchitis, testicular trauma, torsion, tumours, exposure to radiation, chemotherapy, and heat. Other acquired factors are groin surgeries, anti-sperm antibodies, systemic diseases such as liver cirrhosis, varicocele, and erectile dysfunction.

Behavioural factors which affect male fertility include obesity and dietary factors, smoking/vaping, alcohol ingestion, use of recreational drugs and exposure to environmental toxins. These extrinsic factors are often modifiable as they relate to physical activity, environmental exposure, diet, and body habitus. When appropriately controlled, therapy may be achieved and therefore should be the initial step in the management of male infertility. Advanced paternal age is an independent risk factor for poor quality semen and should be considered in the evaluation of male factor infertility especially in the elderly couple. An important extrinsic factor often experienced in rapidly industrialized nations is "stress" which may be physical or psychological. Stress is postulated to negatively affect male fertility due to the associated elevated corticosteroid which suppresses testosterone production and ultimately spermatogenesis [13, 14]. Reactive oxygen species which are by-products of oxygen can be detrimental to semen function as a preponderance of these free radicals over the antioxidant defence mechanism of the body may be injurious to sperm survival [15, 16].

Besides a detailed history and thorough physical examination, the diagnosis of male infertility relies majorly on conventional semen analysis. This is consequent on the fact that normal semen parameters (motility, morphology & count) have been associated with timely reproduction [17, 18]. Furthermore semen analysis is non-invasive and cost effective and it provides in a timely manner the evidence and extent of male contribution to infertility. The latest classification of semen disorders is based on the World Health Organization's (WHO) reference values introduced in 2010 in which semen characteristic threshold for impairments were markedly lowered [19].

4. Investigations

Evaluating male factor infertility begins with a detailed medical history and a comprehensive physical examination. The history seeks to evaluate possible medical causes and risk factors, while the examination aims at providing holistic feedback on the systemic consequences of past exposures and evaluating the current health status of the male partner. During history taking, factors that may affect fertility should be actively sought after such as infectious diseases, genital trauma, groin surgery, diseases in childhood and puberty, exposure to environmental toxins and social/sexual habits. Examination should document body habitus along with the presence or absence of secondary sexual characteristics. A thorough examination of the testis should emphasize size, consistency, presence of masses and symmetry. Varicoceles should be excluded, while a rectal examination is performed to evaluate the prostate gland.

The following are useful investigations in the evaluation of male infertility.

1. Seminal fluid analysis: This is an inexpensive, non-invasive prognostic test of male fertility. Due to wide variability, usually 2 samples are collected 2 weeks apart following 2–5 days of abstinence. Ejaculation occurs preferably in the laboratory into a sterile container. However, for certain psychological reasons, this may be done in a more conducive location such as the patients' home with the aid of the spouse and delivered to the laboratory within 60 minutes of production. Parameters evaluated include semen count, motility, morphology, pH, volume, viscosity, liquefaction time and presence of biochemical markers.

2. Hormone profile: This is very important in distinguishing between obstructive and non-obstructive azoospermia. Very commonly, evaluating follicle-stimulating hormone (FSH), luteinizing hormone (LH) and testosterone will suffice in establishing an endocrine basis for male infertility. More detailed studies are seldomly performed except when indicated.

3. Imaging studies: Ultrasonography is especially important in the assessment of testicular size and evaluation of testicular masses, obstruction, and absence of the vas deferens. It can also be used to evaluate testicular blood floor and reflux in cases of varicocele. The trans-rectal ultrasonography (TRUS) is usually performed in cases of suspected obstruction evidence by seminal volume. Ultrasonography provides an avenue for anatomical evaluation of the male external genitalia with the view to exclude congenital malformations.

4. Semen culture: This is not routinely performed but indicated in the presence of genital tract infections especially following sexually transmitted disease (STD). An increased white cell count in the presence of minimal ejaculate may suggest partial obstruction of the ejaculatory ducts. Spermatotoxic free radicals are increased in the presence of genital infections and may be responsible for diminishing male fertility.

5. Testicular biopsy: A useful diagnostic tool in men with suspected obstructive azoospermia. It is therapeutic during assisted reproductive technique where aspirated/biopsied tissue is teased out to obtain sperm cells which are injected directly into the oocyte via intracytoplasmic sperm injection (ICSI).

6. Sperm DNA fragmentation: is a complimentary test used to evaluate sperm functionality, however its diagnostic accuracy is limited because of lack of discriminatory power especially in predicting outcomes following assisted reproductive technique (ART). There are several tests used to evaluate sperm DNA fragmentation such as sperm chromatin dispersion test (SCD) and sperm chromatin structure assay (SCSA). Infertile men especially oligospermic, obese and alcoholics have been shown to have a higher percentage of fragmented DNA [20].

7. Genetic testing: Certain conditions require genetic testing in the management of male factor infertility, and it has been suggested that the incidence of genetic abnormalities is higher in infertile men requiring assisted reproductive technique. Routine tests recommended for severe semen abnormalities include Y chromosome microdeletion analysis, karyotyping and transmembrane conductance regulator (CFTR) mutation analysis. Fluorescence in situ hybridization technology (FISH) is employed in the direct genetic testing of spermatozoa especially for chromosomal aneuploidy.

5. Management

The management of male factor infertility can sometimes be enigmatic and must take into consideration the presence of concomitant female factors. Generally, management involves lifestyle modification and a combination of either medical or surgical management. Severe male factor infertility will necessitate the deployment of assisted reproductive technology (ART) and in certain instances may require the use of donor sperm especially in the presence of testicular failure. Lifestyle modification through counselling is important in the initial management of alcohol, substance abuse, hazardous occupational exposure, and obesity. A review of medications is quite important since many drugs used in the management of other systemic ailments can affect spermatogenesis.

5.1 Medical management

A variety of hormonal medications have been employed in the medical management of male factor infertility, however, evidence about their efficacy measured by actual pregnancy outcome is questionable [21]. The exception is in the clinical management of gonadotrophin deficiency where replacement with exogenous gonadotrophin is quite effective at enhancing sperm production and conception. In patients with hypogonadotropic hypogonadism, pulsatile gonadotrophin releasing hormone (GnRH) has been found useful and have been associated with improved spermatogenesis. Dopamine agonists such as bromocriptine, cabergoline have been found useful in the management of hyperprolactinaemia. Glucocorticoids on the other hand, have been employed in the successful management of sperm autoimmunity, however the risk of long-term high dose therapy is quite detrimental and early recourse to assisted reproductive technique is preferred. Furthermore, in certain patients with idiopathic oligospermia, tamoxifen, an antioestrogen has been found to increase the rate of natural conception [22]. Antioxidants have been demonstrated to decrease the DNA fragmentation induced by oxidative stress and multivitamin supplementation with vitamins C & E may improve conception [23].

5.2 Surgical management

Several surgical techniques have been employed in the management of male factor infertility with variable outcomes. Varicocelectomy is one of the most performed surgical techniques and it has been demonstrated to improve semen quality in about 44% of those treated [24]. Reconstructive surgical procedures include epididymovasostomy and vasovasostomy which are generally performed as microsurgical procedures. Indications for epididymovasostomy include congenital or acquired obstructions at the level of the epididymis. An important caveat prior to embarking on these procedures is ascertaining testicular function through a hormone profile or testicular biopsy. The development of antisperm antibodies is a limiting factor and this influences pregnancy outcomes in combination with other prognostic factors such as semen quality and age of the female partner.

Obstruction of the prostatic urethra is usually treated by transurethral incision, and this has been demonstrated to improve semen quality and natural conception [25]. Surgical sperm aspiration techniques such as testicular sperm aspiration (TESA), microsurgical epididymal sperm aspiration (MESA) and percutaneous epidydimal sperm aspiration (PESA) are combined with intracytoplasmic sperm injection (ICSI) during assisted reproductive technique in men with obstructive azoospermia. These procedures allow limited spermatozoa to be collected from the male reproductive organ and injected into the oocyte during in-vitro-fertilization (IVF).

5.3 Assisted reproductive technique (ART)

Advancement in the management of infertility has resulted in the deployment of ART which has significantly improved the ability of infertile couples to have their own biologic offspring. This can be achieved using intrauterine insemination (IUI), in-vitro-fertilization (IVF) and intracytoplasmic sperm injection (ICSI). In men with mild semen abnormalities, progressively motile spermatozoa are washed and inseminated during the mid-cycle into the uterine cavity following ovulation induction. However, in the presence of severe semen abnormalities, in-vitro-fertilization, and intracytoplasmic sperm injection (IVF/ICSI) are offered. In men with severe male factor infertility and non-obstructive azoospermia, clinical pregnancy rates following IVF/ICSI have been shown to be lower than men with normospermia, thus demonstrating the importance of careful morphological selection of spermatozoa during ART [26]. Testicular derived spermatozoa have lower amounts of sperm DNA fragmentation compared with ejaculated sperm [27] and it has been suggested albeit cautiously that testicular sperm extraction in combination with ICSI may be beneficial in non-azoospermic men with elevated sperm DNA Fragmentation. Sperm donation should be given consideration in cases of testicular failure.

6. Challenges in developing countries

Male infertility is often relegated to the background in many developing countries and management often focuses on female factors due to deeply rooted sociocultural beliefs and norms. This situation is further compounded by the inequity in access to health facilities and treatment of infertility which is largely uninsured and expensive. There however exist a high premium on childbearing and this inadvertently predisposes infertile couples to seeking alternative and unorthodox care which often result in delays that further worsens the outcome of care. Infertility particularly male factor increases conjugal mobility in a quest to confirm potency and possibly have an offspring. Investigation for male factor infertility is often fraught with resistance and very often only basic tests such as seminal fluid analysis, hormone profile and ultrasonography are readily available. Advanced tests are usually performed at specialized fertility centres which are very few and often concentrated in urban cities.

The cost of assisted conception services is prohibitive and has remained a rate limiting step in the access to advanced fertility care in many developing countries lacking effective health insurance coverage. Furthermore, there exist a preponderance of risk factors ranging from environmental pollution, exposures to occupational hazards, poorly treated sexually transmitted diseases and harmful traditional practices. The panacea for infertility care in developing countries will entail a paradigm shift in perception about aetiology and management through the provision of educational and information services. Efforts must be geared towards the elimination of harmful traditional practices which negatively influence the health seeking behaviour and sometimes pose a risk to compliance with orthodox care. There is also an urgent need to expand the health insurance system such that provision is made for the management of involuntary childlessness. Mitigating risk factors will include the control of environmental pollution and hazard while prioritizing the management and prevention of sexually transmitted diseases. Concerted effort is needed in developing countries to address the gap in access to care through better funding and incorporation of holistic care in the management of male infertility.

7. What does the future hold?

There has been a gradual inclination towards research into protein biomarkers of male infertility, however an important limitation is the lack of unique markers associated with specific medical conditions [28, 29]. It is expected that advancement in disease-targeted sequencing and epigenetic semen analysis will expand the scope of genetic testing and treatment of male infertility [30]. Stem cell therapeutics have witnessed significant improvement and induced pluripotent stem cells have been employed during in-vitro models to produce sperm [31]. It has been suggested that these induced pluripotent stem cells can be utilized with gene editing to correct genetic disorders and restore spermatogenesis in patients who have been exposed to either chemotherapy or radiotherapy [32]. Artificial Intelligence (AI) predictive algorithms have been developed to select men who will benefit from genetic testing and ART [33]. Though in its infancy, the application of AI in andrology and urology seems promising and may be the game changer in the near future [33, 34].

8. Conclusion

Male factor infertility is responsible for about half of the cases of infertility and a sound understanding of the aetiology and treatment options is important for the successful management of involuntary childlessness. In many cases, male infertility is amenable to treatment through lifestyle modifications, medical and surgical interventions and in severe cases, assisted reproductive techniques. Advances in assisted reproductive techniques has offered men who naturally would not be able to conceive the opportunity of having biologic progenies and where testicular failure has been demonstrated, gamete donation or adoption remains a viable option in well motivated couples. Advances in the development of protein biomarkers, stem cell therapeutics and artificial intelligence will further widen the spectrum of therapeutic opportunities available to infertile men (**Figure 1**).

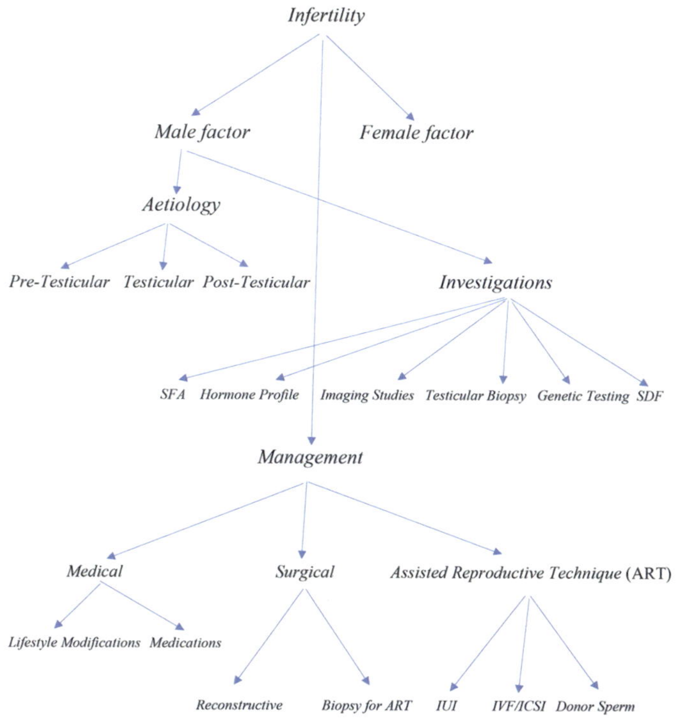

Figure 1.
Schematic representation of the management of male factor infertility. Key: SFA: seminal fluid analysis; SDF: sperm DNA fragmentation; IUI: intrauterine insemination; IVF/ICSI: in-vitro-fertilization/intracytoplasmic sperm injection.

Author details

Gbolahan Oladele Obajimi[1*] and Bamgboye Morakinyo Afolabi[2]

1 Department of Obstetrics and Gynaecology, College of Medicine, University of Ibadan, Nigeria

2 Nigerian Institute of Medical Research, Yaba, Lagos, Nigeria

*Address all correspondence to: gbolahanobajimi@gmail.com

References

[1] WHO. WHO Manual for the Standardized Investigation and Diagnosis of the Infertile Couple. United Kingdom: Cambridge University Press; 2000

[2] Petersen GL, Blenstrup LT, Peterson BD, Knudsen LB, Schmidt L. Impact of childlessness on life and attitudes towards continuation of medically assisted reproduction and/or adoption. Human Fertility Cambridge. Jun 2015;**18**(2):121-127. DOI: 10.3109/14647273.2015.1006691

[3] Wu AK, Elliott P, Katz PP, Smith JF. Time costs of fertility care: The hidden hardship of building a family. Fertility and Sterility. 2013;**99**(7):2025-2030. DOI: 10.1016/j.fertnstert.2013.01.145

[4] Obajimi GO, Kolade CO, Aladejare A. Is male factor infertility rising? Another side of the equation from an in vitro fertilization clinic in southwestern Nigeria. African Journal of Infertility Assistant Concept. 2021;**6**:10-13

[5] Agarwal A, Baskaran S, Parekh N, Cho CL, Henkel R, Vij S, et al. Male infertility. Lancet. 2021;**397**(10271):319-333. DOI: 10.1016/S0140-6736(20)32667-2

[6] Agarwal A, Mulgund A, Hamada A, Chyatte MR. A unique view on male infertility around the globe. Reproductive Biology and Endocrinology. 2015;**13**:37. DOI: 10.1186/s12958-015-0032-1

[7] Krausz C. Male infertility: Pathogenesis and clinical diagnosis. Best Practice & Research. Clinical Endocrinology & Metabolism. 2011;**25**(2):271-285. DOI: 10.1016/j.beem.2010.08.006

[8] Salonia A, Matloob R, Gallina A, Abdollah F, Saccà A, Briganti A, et al. Are infertile men less healthy than fertile men? Results of a prospective case-control survey. European Urology. 2009;**56**(6):1025-1031. DOI: 10.1016/j.eururo.2009.03.001

[9] Hanson BM, Eisenberg ML, Hotaling JM. Male infertility: A biomarker of individual and familial cancer risk. Fertility and Sterility. 2018;**109**(1):6-19. DOI: 10.1016/j.fertnstert.2017.11.005

[10] Gudeloglu A, Parekattil SJ. Update in the evaluation of the azoospermic male. Clinics (Sao Paulo). 2013;**68**(Suppl 1):27-34. DOI: 10.6061/clinics/2013(sup01)04

[11] Craig JR, Jenkins TG, Carrell DT, Hotaling JM. Obesity, male infertility, and the sperm epigenome. Fertility and Sterility. 2017;**107**(4):848-859. DOI: 10.1016/j.fertnstert.2017.02.115

[12] Levine H, Jørgensen N, Martino-Andrade A, Mendiola J, Weksler-Derri D, Mindlis I, et al. Temporal trends in sperm count: A systematic review and meta-regression analysis. Human Reproduction Update. 2017;**23**(6):646-659. DOI: 10.1093/humupd/dmx022

[13] Nargund VH. Effects of psychological stress on male fertility. Nature Reviews. Urology. 2015;**12**(7):373-382. DOI: 10.1038/nrurol.2015.112

[14] Arya ST, Dibb B. The experience of infertility treatment: The male perspective. Human Fertility (Cambridge, England). 2016;**19**(4):242-248. DOI: 10.1080/14647273.2016.1222083

[15] de Lamirande E, Gagnon C. Impact of reactive oxygen species on spermatozoa: A balancing act between beneficial and detrimental effects. Human Reproduction. 1995;**10**(1):15-21

[16] Agarwal A, Prabakaran SA. Mechanism, measurement, and prevention of oxidative stress in male reproductive physiology. Indian Journal of Experimental Biology. 2005;**43**(11):963-974

[17] Esteves SC, Zini A, Aziz N, Alvarez JG, Sabanegh ES Jr, Agarwal A. Critical appraisal of World Health Organization's new reference values for human semen characteristics and effect on diagnosis and treatment of subfertile men. Urology. 2012;**79**(1):16-22. DOI: 10.1016/j.urology.2011.08.003

[18] Agarwal A, Bragais FM, Sabanegh E. Assessing sperm function. The Urologic Clinics of North America. 2008;**35**(2):157-171. DOI: 10.1016/j.ucl.2008.01.012

[19] World Health Organization. WHO Laboratory Manual for the Examination and Processing of Human Semen. 5th ed. Geneva: WHO Press; 2010

[20] Ajayi AB, Afolabi BM, Ajayi VD, Oyetunji IO, Atiba A, Saanu S, et al. Evaluation of Sperm DNA Fragmentation amongst Infertile Black Africans. A Nigerian Study. Open Journal of Urology. 2018;**8**:297-316. DOI: 10.4236/oju.2018.811034

[21] Liu PY, Handelsman DJ. The present and future state of hormonal treatment for male infertility. Human Reproduction Update. 2003;**9**(1):9-23. DOI: 10.1093/humupd/dmg002

[22] Adamopoulos DA, Pappa A, Billa E, Nicopoulou S, Koukkou E, Michopoulos J. Effectiveness of combined tamoxifen citrate and testosterone undecanoate treatment in men with idiopathic oligozoospermia. Fertility and Sterility. 2003;**80**(4):914-920. DOI: 10.1016/s0015-0282(03)01123-3

[23] Makker K, Agarwal A, Sharma R. Oxidative stress and male infertility. The Indian Journal of Medical Research. 2009;**129**(4):357-367

[24] Dohle GR, Colpi GM, Hargreave TB, Papp GK, Jungwirth A. Weidner W; EAU Working Group on Male Infertility. EAU guidelines on male infertility. European Urology. 2005;**48**(5):703-711. DOI: 10.1016/j.eururo.2005.06.002

[25] Schroeder-Printzen I, Ludwig M, Köhn F, Weidner W. Surgical therapy in infertile men with ejaculatory duct obstruction: Technique and outcome of a standardized surgical approach. Human Reproduction. 2000;**15**(6):1364-1368. DOI: 10.1093/humrep/15.6.1364

[26] Lee SH, Song H, Park YS, Koong MK, Song IO, Jun JH. Poor sperm quality affects clinical outcomes of intracytoplasmic sperm injection in fresh and subsequent frozen-thawed cycles: Potential paternal effects on pregnancy outcomes. Fertility and Sterility. 2009;**91**(3):798-804. DOI: 10.1016/j.fertnstert.2007.12.061

[27] Esteves SC, Roque M, Bradley CK, Garrido N. Reproductive outcomes of testicular versus ejaculated sperm for intracytoplasmic sperm injection among men with high levels of DNA fragmentation in semen: Systematic review and meta-analysis. Fertility and Sterility. 2017;**108**(3):456-467. DOI: 10.1016/j.fertnstert.2017.06.018

[28] Swain N, Samanta L, Agarwal A, Kumar S, Dixit A, Gopalan B, et al. Aberrant upregulation of compensatory redox molecular machines may contribute to sperm dysfunction in infertile men with unilateral varicocele: A proteomic insight. Antioxidants & Redox Signaling. 2020;**32**(8):504-521. DOI: 10.1089/ars.2019.7828

[29] Panner Selvam MK, Agarwal A, Pushparaj PN. A quantitative global

proteomics approach to understanding the functional pathways dysregulated in the spermatozoa of asthenozoospermic testicular cancer patients. Andrology. 2019;7(4):454-462. DOI: 10.1111/andr.12620

[30] Thirumavalavan N, Gabrielsen JS, Lamb DJ. Where are we going with gene screening for male infertility? Fertility and Sterility. 2019;**111**(5):842-850. DOI: 10.1016/j.fertnstert.2019.03.036

[31] Nagamatsu G, Hayashi K. Stem cells, *in vitro* gametogenesis and male fertility. Reproduction. 2017;**154**(6):F79-F91. DOI: 10.1530/REP-17-0510

[32] Fang F, Li Z, Zhao Q, Li H, Xiong C. Human induced pluripotent stem cells and male infertility: An overview of current progress and perspectives. Human Reproduction. 2018;**33**(2):188-195. DOI: 10.1093/humrep/dex369

[33] Chu KY, Nassau DE, Arora H, Lokeshwar SD, Madhusoodanan V, Ramasamy R. Artificial intelligence in reproductive urology. Current Urology Reports. 2019;**20**(9):52. DOI: 10.1007/s11934-019-0914-4

[34] Bentellis I, Guérin S, Khene ZE, Khavari R, Peyronnet B. Artificial intelligence in functional urology: How it may shape the future. Current Opinion in Urology. 2021;**31**(4):385-390. DOI: 10.1097/MOU.0000000000000888

Chapter 2

Advances in Epigenetic Mechanisms and Transgenerational Inheritance of Male Infertility Induced by Exposure to Endocrine-Disrupting Chemicals

Yan Yuan, Peihao Wu, Yixuan Yan, Jing Wang, Jialin Feng, Jinqi Ma, Qiuqin Tang and Wei Wu

Abstract

Male fertility has declined over the last few decades. Therefore, the increasing concern about the link between the environment and male reproductive health has been raised. Studies have found that the exposure to environmental toxicants during fetal development or the mother's perinatal period promotes the occurrence of infertility in adult male offspring. Environmental toxicants, especially endocrine disrupting chemicals (EDCs), such as phthalic acid ester (PAEs), can induce changes in epigenetic information related to paternal infertility, threatening the reproductive, and developmental health of offspring. Transgenerational epigenetic inheritance refers to a genetic phenomenon that does not involve DNA sequences and affects the phenotypic characteristics of offspring by altering gene expression through DNA or RNA methylation, histone modification, noncoding RNAs, etc. This review describes the concept and phenotype of intergenerational and transgenerational inheritance induced by EDCs, summarizes the recent achievements of important epigenetic molecular mechanisms, and provides a relevant theoretical basis for the protection of male fertility.

Keywords: transgenerational inheritance, endocrine disrupting chemicals, male infertility, DNA methylation, m^6A modification

1. Introduction

At least 180 million couples worldwide are affected by infertility, with male factors accounting for approximately 50% [1]. Levine et al. found through a meta-analysis that during the decades from 1973 to 2011, there was a significant decrease in sperm count among males from North America, Europe, and Australia, with no trend toward remission [2]. They further explored and found that such a phenomenon also existed in males from South America, Asia, and Africa. The declining trend continues and has become even steeper since 2000 [3]. The findings above strongly indicate that there has been a significant decline in male reproductive health in the past 50 years, leading to significant fertility issues that cannot be ignored.

Many factors can cause male infertility, mainly known as Klinefelter syndrome, varicocele, environmental or occupational exposure to toxic chemicals [4], heavy metals [5, 6], smoking [7] and drinking [8], etc. Experimental and epidemiological studies show a strong connection between exposure to environmental endocrine-disrupting chemicals (EDCs) and impaired male fertility [9–11]. EDCs refer to "an exogenous chemical substance released into the environment due to human production or life, interfering with hormone action in humans and animals," which damage the homeostasis of the endocrine system by inhibiting or promoting hormone production, secretion [12] and transport [13, 14] in the body, which raise a worldwide public health concern [15, 16].

Exposure to EDCs during pregnancy will lead to damage to testicular function, spermatogenesis disorder, and fertility decline of offspring [17]. EDCs, such as bisphenol A (BPA), enhance susceptibility to diseases, especially male reproductive system diseases [18], which are significantly correlated with epigenetic variations [19]. Epigenetics refer to the mechanism by which genetic information of related traits is transmitted to offspring through DNA or RNA methylation, histone modification, noncoding RNA, and so on, without changing DNA sequences [20]. Obvious abnormality of DNA and histone methylation (e.g., H3K4me and H3K27me) can be observed in the sperm of men with reproductive disorders [21].

Changes in epigenetic information caused by ancestral exposure can still be transmitted to offspring without direct exposure to environmental factors, which is known as epigenetic transgenerational inheritance [22, 23]. Yuan et al. found that there was a decline in the number of sperm and Sertoli cells in the generations, from F1 to F3, of male Sprague–Dawley rats whose ancestral female rats (F0) were exposed to BPA during pregnancy [24].

When it comes to transgenerational inheritance, it is necessary to define phenotype to make a distinction between direct exposure effects and germ-cell-mediated transgenerational effects [25]. Take EDCs exposure for example. If the pregnant female (F0) is exposed to EDCs, the developing embryo (F1) and the germ cells (F2) that have occurred in the embryo are also directly exposed to EDCs. Therefore, the first generation which is not directly exposed to EDCs is the F3 generation. If the nonpregnant female (F0) is exposed to EDCs, the germ cells that produce the F1 generation are also directly exposed to EDCs, while the F2 generation is not directly exposed to EDCs [21, 23]. In both cases above, postnatal exposure assessment should be conducted for F3 or F2 to identify transgenerational inheritance.

2. Epigenetic mechanism

2.1 DNA methylation

DNA methylation is one of the important epigenetic modifications in cells. Due to the semi-reserved nature of DNA replication, the DNA methylation pattern on the parent chain can be replicated on the newly synthesized subchain, realizing the inheritance of DNA methylation [26]. It was found that abnormal sperm DNA methylation was negatively correlated with semen quality, spermatogenesis, and male fertility [27]. In eukaryotes, DNA methyltransferases (Dnmts), which promote and maintain DNA methylation [28], and coregulate gene expression with demethylase

TET dioxygenase [29], catalyze the methylation of cytosine at C5 to form 5-methylcytosine (5mC), the main form of DNA methylation [30]. 5mC is a stable epigenetic marker of transcriptional inhibition in gene enhancers and promoters.

The key feature of DNA methylation is the symmetrical 5mC modification of CpG dinucleotide [31], usually found in the promotor of DNA, where methylation causes gene silencing [27]. The region with high sequences of CpG is called CpG island (CGI). Imprinted genes can still retain the methylation pattern of parental allele after global genome demethylation after fertilization [27]. Song et al. found that poor semen parameters, which can prompt semen quality, were highly related to abnormal methylation at some CpG sites of imprinted genes, including spermatogenesis disorder and severe damage to DNA integrity [32].

A recent research conducted by Takahashi et al., based on the completion of CGI-targeted methylation on metabolic-related genes (Ankrd26 and Ldlr) of embryonic stem cells (ESCs) in mice, found that DNA methylation-edited mice showed abnormal metabolic phenotype, and this acquired methylation could be passed on in offspring [33]. The author inserted a DNA fragment that is free of the CpG site into the CGI near promotor to induce de novo DNA methylation of the CGI. When the DNA fragment was removed, the state and level of the methylation remained unchanged in the offspring mice, resistant to demethylation after fertilization [34, 35].

Thorson et al. explored the transgenerational effects of pesticides on the male reproductive ability by constructing a pesticide (permethrin and DEET combination) infected mouse model. They found that if the pregnant female (F0) was exposed to pesticides, abnormal spermatogenetic phenomena such as atrophy of seminiferous tubule and spermatogenic arrest, were observed in the testis of both F1 and F3 generation, as well as specific differentially methylated regions (DMRs) in sperm [36]. Consistently, exposure of the F0 female mice to p,p'-DDE during pregnancy led to changes in DNA methylation levels of H19 and Gtl2 in the sperm of the F1 male mice, which was transferred to the F3 generation through the paternal germ line [37].

The findings above highly demonstrate that the DNA methylation pattern can be transferred across generations through the parental germ line.

2.2 RNA methylation

N6-methyladenosine (m^6A) is generated after methylation at the 6th nitrogen atom of adenine, which is the most common endogenous posttranscriptional modification (PTM) of mRNA in eukaryotes [38], affecting cycle stages of mRNA from processing, output, translation to degradation [38, 39]. The m^6A modification occurs on various RNAs, including protein-coding transcripts, like mRNAs, tRNAs, and rRNAs, and noncoding RNAs, like lncRNAs [40].

The biological function of m^6A modification is mediated by methyltransferase, demethylase, and binding proteins, dynamically and reversibly [41, 42]. The imbalance of m^6A modification is related to spermatogenesis disorder and infertility in males [43]. A recent study found that FTO, a demethylase, regulated testosterone receptor AR dependent on m^6A, affecting the maturation of Leydig cells and spermatogenesis [44].

Chen Y et al. observed that m^6A methylation affected the transcriptional stability of CAMKK2β, a calcium-dependent protein kinase that suppressed AMP-activated protein kinase (AMPK) and the translation of PPM1A, a magnesium-dependent protein phosphatase that promoted AMPK expression to modulate autophagy, thereby regulating testosterone synthesis in Leydig cells. As well, a significant decline of m^6A methylation was observed in Leydig cells from patients with oligospermia or azoospermia [45]. The research indicated that m^6A methylation had important implications for male reproductive health.

Research has shown that injecting sperm tsRNAs from high-fat diet mice into normal zygote would cause metabolic disorder in offspring, suggesting that paternal phenotypes can be transmitted across generations through sperm tsRNAs [46]. But, this effect disappeared in $Dnmt2^{-/-}$ mice. Simultaneously, RNA methylation levels significantly decreased, leading to changes in the structure and function of tsRNAs, which pointed out the importance of RNA methylation in the occurrence of transgenerational inheritance [47]. However, the role of m^6A modification in the epigenetic transgenerational inheritance of male infertility has not been elucidated, and further research is needed.

2.3 Histone modification

Chromatin carries genetic information and consists of nucleosome and histones, which includes H2A, H2B, H3, and H4 [48]. Environmental factors can affect the density of chromatin or signal transduction of transcription factors by inducing posttranslational modifications (PTMs) of histones [49], which are often referred to as epigenetic marks, including methylation, phosphorylation, acetylation, ubiquitination, etc., to regulate chromatin structure and gene expression [50, 51].

In most species, lysine methylation is the frequent form of histone modification. Chromatin inhibition is related to the enrichment of H3 lysine 9 trimethylation (H3K9me3) [52] and H3 lysine 27 trimethylation (H3K27me3) [53], while H3 lysine 4 trimethylation (H3K4me3) [54] peaking around the transcriptional start site (TSS) produces a marked effect in the process of the initiation of transcription [55]. It was found that the inhibition of H3K4 methylation during spermatogenesis, possibly related to the decrease of transcriptional activity of developing sperm, led to developmental defects and health damage of offspring, which was transmitted paternally for three generations, indicating that epigenetic modification of sperm has an impact on the health of offspring [56, 57].

Histone modification is jointly regulated by lysine methyltransferase (KMT) enzymes and demethylase (KDM) enzymes, identifying methylation sites through binding proteins to participate in various biological processes [58]. Ribeiro et al. found that GCNA, a histone-binding protein whose mutations in locus were responsible for azoospermia in men [59], played a crucial role in long-term spermatogenesis [60]. It was reported that H3K4me3 was involved in the formation of double-strand breaks (DSBs) during the meiosis of spermatogonium, which is related to spermatogenesis. In this process, Cfp1, a component of KDM enzymes, is dynamically expressed to protect meiosis [61].

An animal experiment carried out by Skinner et al. showed that being exposed to DDT, a kind of EDCs, during the pregnancy of female mice (F0) was responsible for the alteration of H3K27me3 methylation level in the sperm of the F3 male mice, generating apoptosis of testicular germ cells, which was linked to differential histone retention regions (DHRs). However, it was not observed in the F1 or F2 generation [62]. This suggested the critical role of histone modification in the transgenerational inheritance induced by EDCs.

2.4 Noncoding RNAs

Noncoding RNAs (ncRNAs) refer to RNAs that do not participate in encoding proteins, including small noncoding RNAs (sncRNAs), which cover microRNAs (miRNAs), small interfering RNAs (siRNAs), etc., long noncoding RNAs (lncRNAs) and circular RNAs (circRNAs), etc. [63]. NcRNAs are involved in mediating cellular biological processes, including gene expression, PTMs, and signal transduction, regulating individual development and disease [64, 65].

In eukaryotic cells, ncRNAs modulate various physiological processes, including spermatogenesis and spermatozoa maturation, by up or down-regulating gene expression [66]. Research showed that reduced expression of miR-525-3p was related to poor sperm quantity, quality, and morphology in patients with asthenozoospermia [67].

Recently, the effect of sperm sncRNAs in regulating early life development and epigenetic inheritance has been focused on. It makes transgenerational inheritance possible that sncRNAs mediate other epigenetic mechanisms, like DNA methylation and histone modifications [68]. Liu et al. found that sperm sncRNAs, including tsRNAs and rsRNAs, provided support for the transgenerational inheritance of paternal metabolic disorder phenotype [69].

It was reported that prenatal dexamethasone exposure resulted in changes in testicular morphology, with the decrease of Leydig cells and the inhibition of testosterone production in offspring male mice, consistent with the effect of the F3 generation. Liu et al. discovered that the expression of miR-466b-3p declined in sperm of both F1 and F3 male mice, which indicated that miR-466b-3p may mediate the transgenerational effects of reproductive toxicity induced by dexamethasone [70].

CircRNAs are found in human testis, sperm, and seminal plasma while studied limitedly, making it a novel object in the field of male reproduction. It was reported that circRNAs may be associated with sperm quality control [71], DNA replication, cell cycle, and meiosis [72]. A significant difference was observed between the expression level of circRNAs in the sperm of asthenozoospermic patients and normozoospermic males [73].

3. Transgenerational inheritance induced by EDCs

3.1 Phthalic acid esters (PAEs)

Plastics are widely used in daily life, exposed through Inhalation, ingestion, and dermal absorption [74]. PAEs, such as di (2-ethylhexyl) phthalate (DEHP) and dibutyl phthalate (DBP), are frequently-used plasticizers in plastic products, which have teratogenicity, carcinogenicity, mutagenicity, and reproductive toxicity, posing a serious threat to human reproductive and developmental health [75].

An epidemiological study found that PAE exposure was associated with a decrease in male reproductive quality [76, 77]. Yang et al. discovered that in adolescent SD rats, DEHP inhibited the expression of Sod2, Igf-1, and Gpx1 by upregulating the methylation level of the CpG sites around promotor regions, resulting in injury of testis, including decreased serum testosterone level, apoptosis of spermatogenic cells, dysfunction of Leydig cells, etc. [78]. Another research came to the consistent conclusion that DEHP exposure reduced the expression of antioxidant indicators in testes, such as Cat, Sod1, Prdx6, and Sirt1, thus increasing the production of reactive oxygen species (ROS), which significantly affected the proliferation of germ cells, leading to poor sperm quality and male infertility [79].

The phenotype of male reproductive disorders caused by PAEs exposure can be passed on to offspring through the paternal germ line. Doyle et al. found that the morphology of the testicular seminiferous tubule of male offspring, from the F1 generation to the F4 generation, whose female ancestry was exposed to DEHP during pregnancy was abnormal; meanwhile, the sperm count and motility of male offspring were reduced. Damage to the function of spermatogonial stem cells (SSCs) was also found in the F3 generation [80].

The exact molecular mechanism of the transgenerational inheritance of the function disruption in germ cells and SSCs remains unclear, but there have been articles indicating that disease-specific DMR is found in the sperm of the F3 male rats [81]. It was reported that gestational exposure to DEHP led to impaired male reproductive function and increased DNA fragmentation index (DFI) across generations. Hsu et al. discovered in the F3 generation that compared to the control group, DMRs were observed in all DEHP exposure groups, with more in the group which was highly exposed [82].

3.2 Bisphenol a (BPA)

BPA is an industrial plasticizer that is widely consumed [83] with estrogenic activity, which can bind to androgen receptors and act as an antagonist to block the function of endogenous androgen [84]. The study found that increased BPA concentration in male urine was significantly related to spermatogenesis disorder and poor semen quality [85]. BPA has a transgenerational impact on the reproductive ability of offspring [86] by affecting sperm epigenetic modulations, including improving global DNA-specific CpG site methylation and decreasing histone modifications [87].

Ryu et al. found that BPA caused the elevation of H3 modification and DNA methylation in the testis, affecting the expression level of core histones, which interfered with the transformation from histone to protamine during spermatogenesis, thus leading to spermatogenesis disorder and fertility decline [88]. An experiment conducted on zebrafish also confirmed the conclusion that BPA caused male infertility. González-Rojo et al. found that BPA led to a rise in the activity of histone acetyltransferase, increasing the acetylation level of histones (H3K9ac, H3K14ac and H4K12ac). What is more, the acetylation effect can be transmitted across generations paternally [89].

Animal toxicity experiments are often limited to exposure to individual toxic substances. An epidemiological study investigated the relationship between bisphenol A and its analogs in urine and semen quality [90]. It was found that high BPA exposure was negatively correlated with semen concentration, sperm count, and motility, while high BPS exposure was negatively correlated with sperm motility. When bisphenol mixtures were more than 55th percentiles, the impairment of semen quality was also observed.

3.3 Per- and polyfluoroalkyl substances (PFAS)

Per- and poly-fluoroalkyl substances (PFAS) are a kind of organic compound mainly composed of carbon and fluorine atoms, which are widely used in textiles, surfactants, food packaging, and other fields. However, because of their high thermal stability and chemical stability, they can persist in the environment and not be biodegraded [91]. PFAS exposure is associated with multiple adverse outcomes, including reproductive and developmental toxicity [92].

It was found that high exposure to perfluorinated compounds (PFCs) led to male gonadal dysplasia, decreased sperm count and semen quality, and increased infertility, as well as lower levels of testosterone and proliferation of Leydig cells [93–95].

The reproductive toxicity caused by PFAS exposure is related to changes in membrane permeability, disruption of mitochondrial function, disruption of blood-testis barrier (BTB), decreased gonadotropin-releasing hormone (GnRH) secretion, and so on [96].

There has been no literature report on the transgenerational inheritance of PFAS reproductive toxicity. This is a gap and challenge in the field of male reproduction. Strict research is still needed in the future.

4. Discussion

This review summarizes the epigenetic mechanisms and transgenerational inheritance of male infertility caused by environmental endocrine-disrupting chemicals. In the field of male reproduction, DNA methylation, histone modification, and noncoding RNAs have been studied relatively thoroughly, although people seem to be more interested in the molecular biological mechanism which mediates toxicological reactions occurred in offspring.

Like methylation, acetylation, and ubiquitination, SUMOylation as a kind of post-transcriptional modification has gradually attracted attention and research, which is reported that mediates the localization and function of target proteins by binding to them [97]. SUMOylation regulates chromatin structure and gene expression by PTMs on histones [98]. Nowadays, few researchers have associated SUMOylation with male reproduction, let alone the transgenerational inheritance of phenotypes of reproductive disorders. This may be an innovation of research in the field of reproduction in the future.

NcRNAs make it possible for transgenerational gene regulation [68]. There is clear evidence in cancers that lncRNAs can mediate DNA methylation in both physiological and pathological conditions, as well as histone modifications and chromatin remodeling, regulating various transcription processes [99]. Similarly, it is found that PIWI-interacting RNAs (piRNAs) mediate de novo DNA methylation in paternal germ cells [100]. However, few researchers have combined ncRNAs with other epigenetic mechanisms to explain the occurrence of related phenotypes in male infertility.

Although significant progress has been made in the research on the basic mechanism of transgenerational inheritance, the relationship between epigenetics and environmental exposure is still unclear, and most of them are carried out in animals. Therefore, it is not clear whether there is a similar mechanism in humans. Combining population data with animal experiments can promote research on the transgenerational inheritance of male reproductive disorders induced by EDCs.

The results of existing research findings show that many reproductive diseases and infertility today may be partially mediated by environmental exposure to ancestry across generations [101]. Genetic factors and heritability should be taken into consideration in the risk assessment of reproductive diseases, and relevant epigenetic markers should be used to assist in diagnosis to prevent or reduce the occurrence of diseases.

5. Conclusions

This review summarizes the recent achievements of important epigenetic molecular mechanisms, such as DNA or RNA methylation, histone modification, ncRNAs, and transgenerational inheritance induced by environmental endocrine-disrupting chemicals, such as PAEs, BPA, and PFAS. In this review, the transgenerational epigenetic phenotype is clearly defined. At the same time, it is proposed to combine ncRNAs with other epigenetic mechanisms to explain the mechanism of transgenerational inheritance of male infertility.

Acknowledgements

This work was supported by the National Key Project of Research and Development Program (2022YFC2702902), National Natural Science Foundation of China (82273662, 81971405), Jiangsu Natural Science Foundation (BK20221307), Major Project of Natural Science Research in Jiangsu Province Colleges and Universities (20KJA330001), Medical Research Project of Jiangsu Health and Health Commission (Z2019010), the Major Research plan of the National Natural Science Foundation of China (91943301), and the Priority Academic Program for the Development of Jiangsu Higher Education Institutions (Public Health and Preventive Medicine).

Conflict of interest

The authors declare no conflict of interest.

Author details

Yan Yuan[1,2], Peihao Wu[1,2], Yixuan Yan[1,2], Jing Wang[1,2], Jialin Feng[1,2], Jinqi Ma[3], Qiuqin Tang[4*] and Wei Wu[1,2*]

1 State Key Laboratory of Reproductive Medicine, Wuxi Medical Center, School of Public Health, Nanjing Medical University, Nanjing, China

2 Key Laboratory of Modern Toxicology of Ministry of Education, School of Public Health, Nanjing Medical University, Nanjing, China

3 The Affiliated Wuxi People's Hospital of Nanjing Medical University, Wuxi People's Hospital, Wuxi Medical Center, Nanjing Medical University, Nanjing, China

4 Department of Obstetrics, Women's Hospital of Nanjing Medical University, Nanjing Maternity and Child Health Care Hospital, Nanjing, China

*Address all correspondence to: tqq19871004@126.com and wwu@njmu.edu.cn

References

[1] Leslie SW, Soon-Sutton TL, Khan MAB. Male Infertility. Treasure Island (FL): StatPearls Publishing; 2023

[2] Levine H et al. Temporal trends in sperm count: A systematic review and meta-regression analysis. Human Reproduction Update. 2017;**23**(6):646-659

[3] Levine H et al. Temporal trends in sperm count: A systematic review and meta-regression analysis of samples collected globally in the 20th and 21st centuries. Human Reproduction Update. 2023;**29**(2):157-176

[4] Agarwal A et al. Male infertility. Lancet (London, England). 2021;**397**(10271):319-333

[5] Goutam Mukherjee A et al. Heavy metal and metalloid - induced reproductive toxicity. Environmental Toxicology and Pharmacology. 2022;**92**:103859

[6] Li R-Y et al. Heavy metal ions exchange driven protein phosphorylation cascade functions in genomic instability in spermatocytes and male infertility. Nucleic Acids Research. 2023;**51**(7):3150-3165

[7] Tang Q et al. Semen quality and cigarette smoking in a cohort of healthy fertile men. Environmental Epidemiology (Philadelphia, Pa.). 2019;**3**(4):e055

[8] Basic M et al. Tobacco and alcohol as factors for male infertility-a public health approach. Journal of Public Health (Oxford, England). 2022;**45**(2):e241-e249

[9] Rodprasert W, Toppari J, Virtanen HE. Environmental toxicants and male fertility. Best Practice & Research. Clinical Obstetrics & Gynaecology. 2023;**86**:102298

[10] Guerra MT et al. Reproductive toxicity of maternal exposure to di(2-ethylhexyl)phthalate and butyl paraben (alone or in association) on both male and female Wistar offspring. Journal of Applied Toxicology: JAT. 2023;**43**(2):242-261

[11] Smarr MM et al. Preconception seminal plasma concentrations of endocrine disrupting chemicals in relation to semen quality parameters among male partners planning for pregnancy. Environmental Research. 2018;**167**:78-86

[12] Goktepe O et al. The effect of different doses of nonylphenol on the blood-testicular barrier integrity, hormone level, and DNA damage in the testes of rats. Food and Chemical Toxicology. 2023;**177**:113816

[13] Virant-Klun I, Imamovic-Kumalic S, Pinter B. From oxidative stress to male infertility: Review of the associations of endocrine-disrupting chemicals (Bisphenols, phthalates, and parabens) with human semen quality. Antioxidants (Basel, Switzerland). 2022;**11**(8):1617

[14] Ahn C, Jeung E-B. Endocrine-disrupting chemicals and disease endpoints. International Journal of Molecular Sciences. 2023;**24**(6):5342

[15] Gore AC. Endocrine-disrupting chemicals. JAMA Internal Medicine. 2016;**176**(11):1705-1706

[16] Yilmaz B et al. Endocrine disrupting chemicals: Exposure, effects on human health, mechanism of action, models

for testing and strategies for prevention. Reviews in Endocrine & Metabolic Disorders. 2020;**21**(1):127-147

[17] Green MP et al. Endocrine disrupting chemicals: Impacts on human fertility and fecundity during the peri-conception period. Environmental Research. 2021;**194**:110694

[18] Yadav SK et al. Susceptibility of male reproductive system to bisphenol a, an endocrine disruptor: Updates from epidemiological and experimental evidence. Journal of Biochemical and Molecular Toxicology. 2023;**37**(4):e23292

[19] Sang Q, Ray PF, Wang L. Understanding the genetics of human infertility. Science (New York, N.Y.). 2023;**380**(6641):158-163

[20] Harvey ZH, Chen Y, Jarosz DF. Protein-based inheritance: Epigenetics beyond the chromosome. Molecular Cell. 2018;**69**(2):195-202

[21] Fitz-James MH, Cavalli G. Molecular mechanisms of transgenerational epigenetic inheritance. Nature Reviews. Genetics. 2022;**23**(6):325-341

[22] Legoff L et al. Transgenerational inheritance of environmentally induced epigenetic alterations during mammalian development. Cell. 2019;**8**(12):1559

[23] Guerrero-Bosagna C, Skinner MK. Environmentally induced epigenetic transgenerational inheritance of male infertility. Current Opinion in Genetics & Development. 2014;**26**:79-88

[24] Yuan B et al. From the cover: Metabolomics reveals a role of betaine in prenatal DBP exposure-induced epigenetic transgenerational failure of spermatogenesis in rats. Toxicological Sciences. 2017;**158**(2):356-366

[25] Skinner MK. What is an epigenetic transgenerational phenotype? F3 or F2. Reproductive Toxicology (Elmsford, N.Y.). 2008;**25**(1):2-6

[26] O'Brown ZK, Greer EL. N6-Methyladenine: A conserved and dynamic DNA mark. Advances in Experimental Medicine and Biology. 2016;**945**:213-246

[27] Rotondo JC et al. Epigenetics of male infertility: The role of DNA methylation. Frontiers in Cell and Developmental Biology. 2021;**9**:689624

[28] Castillo-Aguilera O et al. DNA methylation targeting: The DNMT/HMT crosstalk challenge. Biomolecules. 2017;7(1):3

[29] Wu X, Zhang Y. TET-mediated active DNA demethylation: Mechanism, function and beyond. Nature Reviews. Genetics. 2017;**18**(9):517-534

[30] Liberman N, Wang SY, Greer EL. Transgenerational epigenetic inheritance: From phenomena to molecular mechanisms. Current Opinion in Neurobiology. 2019;**59**:189-206

[31] Breiling A, Lyko F. Epigenetic regulatory functions of DNA modifications: 5-methylcytosine and beyond. Epigenetics & Chromatin. 2015;**8**:24

[32] Song B et al. Poor semen parameters are associated with abnormal methylation of imprinted genes in sperm DNA. Reproductive Biology and Endocrinology: RB&E. 2022;**20**(1):155

[33] Takahashi Y et al. Transgenerational inheritance of acquired epigenetic signatures at CpG islands in mice. Cell. 2023;**186**(4):715-731.e19

[34] Horsthemke B, Bird A. Loss of CpG island immunity to DNA methylation

induced by mutation. Epigenetics & Chromatin. 2023;**16**(1):17

[35] Burgess DJ. Engineering transgenerational epigenetic inheritance in mammals. Nature Reviews. Genetics. 2023;**24**(4):209

[36] Thorson JLM et al. Epigenome-wide association study for pesticide (permethrin and DEET) induced DNA methylation epimutation biomarkers for specific transgenerational disease. Environmental Health: a Global Access Science Source. 2020;**19**(1):109

[37] Song Y, Yang L. Transgenerational impaired spermatogenesis with sperm H19 and Gtl2 hypomethylation induced by the endocrine disruptor p,p'-DDE. Toxicology Letters. 2018;**297**:34-41

[38] An Y, Duan H. The role of m6A RNA methylation in cancer metabolism. Molecular Cancer. 2022;**21**(1):14

[39] Sun T, Wu R, Ming L. The role of m6A RNA methylation in cancer. Biomedicine & Pharmacotherapy = Biomedecine & Pharmacotherapie. 2019;**112**:108613

[40] Liu Y et al. LncRNA-PACERR induces pro-tumour macrophages via interacting with miR-671-3p and m6A-reader IGF2BP2 in pancreatic ductal adenocarcinoma. Journal of Hematology & Oncology. 2022;**15**(1):52

[41] Wang J-Y, Lu A-Q. The biological function of m6A reader YTHDF2 and its role in human disease. Cancer Cell International. 2021;**21**(1):109

[42] Sendinc E, Shi Y. RNA m6A methylation across the transcriptome. Molecular Cell. 2023;**83**(3):428-441

[43] Cai Z, Niu Y, Li H. RNA N6-methyladenosine modification, spermatogenesis, and human male infertility. Molecular Human Reproduction. 2021;**27**(6):gaab020

[44] Wu Y et al. Fat mass and obesity-associated factor (FTO)-mediated N6-methyladenosine regulates spermatogenesis in an age-dependent manner. The Journal of Biological Chemistry. 2023;**299**:104783

[45] Chen Y et al. mA mRNA methylation regulates testosterone synthesis through modulating autophagy in Leydig cells. Autophagy. 2021;**17**(2):457-475

[46] Chen Q et al. Sperm tsRNAs contribute to intergenerational inheritance of an acquired metabolic disorder. Science (New York, N.Y.). 2016;**351**(6271):397-400

[47] Zhang Y et al. Dnmt2 mediates intergenerational transmission of paternally acquired metabolic disorders through sperm small non-coding RNAs. Nature Cell Biology. 2018;**20**(5):535-540

[48] Lai WKM, Pugh BF. Understanding nucleosome dynamics and their links to gene expression and DNA replication. Nature Reviews. Molecular Cell Biology. 2017;**18**(9):548-562

[49] Bannister AJ, Kouzarides T. Regulation of chromatin by histone modifications. Cell Research. 2011;**21**(3):381-395

[50] Millán-Zambrano G et al. Histone post-translational modifications - cause and consequence of genome function. Nature Reviews. Genetics. 2022;**23**(9):563-580

[51] Katan-Khaykovich Y, Struhl K. Splitting of H3-H4 tetramers at transcriptionally active genes undergoing dynamic histone exchange. Proceedings of the National Academy of Sciences

of the United States of America. 2011;**108**(4):1296-1301

[52] Ninova M, Fejes Tóth K, Aravin AA. The control of gene expression and cell identity by H3K9 trimethylation. Development (Cambridge, England). 2019;**146**(19):dev181180

[53] Riising EM et al. Gene silencing triggers polycomb repressive complex 2 recruitment to CpG islands genome wide. Molecular Cell. 2014;**55**(3):347-360

[54] Hörmanseder E et al. H3K4 methylation-dependent memory of somatic cell identity inhibits reprogramming and development of nuclear transfer embryos. Cell Stem Cell. 2017;**21**(1):135-143.e6

[55] Black JC, Van Rechem C, Whetstine JR. Histone lysine methylation dynamics: Establishment, regulation, and biological impact. Molecular Cell. 2012;**48**(4):491-507

[56] Siklenka K et al. Disruption of histone methylation in developing sperm impairs offspring health transgenerationally. Science (New York, N.Y.). 2015;**350**(6261):aab2006

[57] Lismer A et al. Histone H3 lysine 4 trimethylation in sperm is transmitted to the embryo and associated with diet-induced phenotypes in the offspring. Developmental Cell. 2021;**56**(5): 671-686.e6

[58] Hyun K et al. Writing, erasing and reading histone lysine methylations. Experimental & Molecular Medicine. 2017;**49**(4):e324

[59] Hardy JJ et al. Variants in GCNA, X-linked germ-cell genome integrity gene, identified in men with primary spermatogenic failure. Human Genetics. 2021;**140**(8):1169-1182

[60] Ribeiro J, Crossan GP. GCNA is a histone binding protein required for spermatogonial stem cell maintenance. Nucleic Acids Research. 2023;**51**(10):4791-4813

[61] Ki BS et al. Epigenetic regulator Cfp1 safeguards male meiotic progression by regulating meiotic gene expression. Experimental & Molecular Medicine. 2022;**54**(8):1098-1108

[62] Skinner MK et al. Alterations in sperm DNA methylation, non-coding RNA and histone retention associate with DDT-induced epigenetic transgenerational inheritance of disease. Epigenetics & Chromatin. 2018;**11**(1):8

[63] Matera AG, Terns RM, Terns MP. Non-coding RNAs: Lessons from the small nuclear and small nucleolar RNAs. Nature Reviews. Molecular Cell Biology. 2007;**8**(3):209-220

[64] Anastasiadou E, Jacob LS, Slack FJ. Non-coding RNA networks in cancer. Nature Reviews. Cancer. 2018;**18**(1):5-18

[65] Slack FJ, Chinnaiyan AM. The role of non-coding RNAs in oncology. Cell. 2019;**179**(5):1033-1055

[66] Barbu MG et al. The roles of MicroRNAs in male infertility. International Journal of Molecular Sciences. 2021;**22**(6):2910

[67] Zhou QZ et al. Expressions of miR-525-3p and its target gene SEMG1 in the spermatozoa of patients with asthenozoospermia. Andrology. 2019;**7**(2):220-227

[68] Yang C et al. Role of small RNAs harbored by sperm in embryonic development and offspring phenotype. Andrology. 2023;**11**(4):770-782

[69] Liu J et al. Paternal phthalate exposure-elicited offspring metabolic disorders are associated with altered sperm small RNAs in mice. Environment International. 2023;**172**:107769

[70] Liu Y et al. MiR-466b-3p/HDAC7 meditates transgenerational inheritance of testicular testosterone synthesis inhibition induced by prenatal dexamethasone exposure. Biochemical Pharmacology. 2022;**199**:115018

[71] Chioccarelli T et al. Expression patterns of circular RNAs in high quality and poor quality human spermatozoa. Frontiers in Endocrinology. 2019;**10**:435

[72] Lin X et al. Expression dynamics, relationships, and transcriptional regulations of diverse transcripts in mouse spermatogenic cells. RNA Biology. 2016;**13**(10):1011-1024

[73] Manfrevola F et al. CircRNA role and circRNA-dependent network (ceRNET) in Asthenozoospermia. Frontiers in Endocrinology. 2020;**11**:395

[74] Huang S et al. A critical review on human internal exposure of phthalate metabolites and the associated health risks. Environmental Pollution (Barking, Essex: 1987). 2021;**279**:116941

[75] Zhang Y et al. Hazards of phthalates (PAEs) exposure: A review of aquatic animal toxicology studies. The Science of the Total Environment. 2021;**771**:145418

[76] Cosci I et al. Lipophilic phthalic acid esters impair human sperm acrosomal reaction through the likely inhibition of phospholipase A2-signaling pathway. Biochemical Pharmacology. 2022;**205**:115249

[77] Bloom MS et al. Associations between urinary phthalate concentrations and semen quality parameters in a general population. Human Reproduction (Oxford, England). 2015;**30**(11):2645-2657

[78] Yang L et al. DEHP-induced testicular injury through gene methylation pathway and the protective effect of soybean isoflavones in Sprague-Dawley rats. Chemico-Biological Interactions. 2021;**348**:109569

[79] XueXia L et al. Di-2-ethylhexyl phthalate (DEHP) exposure induces sperm quality and functional defects in mice. Chemosphere. 2023;**312**(Pt 1):137216

[80] Doyle TJ et al. Transgenerational effects of di-(2-ethylhexyl) phthalate on testicular germ cell associations and spermatogonial stem cells in mice. Biology of Reproduction. 2013;**88**(5):112

[81] Thorson JLM et al. Ancestral plastics exposure induces transgenerational disease-specific sperm epigenome-wide association biomarkers. Environmental. Epigenetics. 2021;**7**(1):dvaa023

[82] Hsu P-C et al. Transgenerational effects of Di(2-Ethylhexyl) phthalate on Anogenital distance, sperm functions and DNA methylation in rat offspring. International Journal of Molecular Sciences. 2021;**22**(8):4131

[83] Mashay Al-Anazi K et al. Maternal and developmental toxicity of Bisphenol-a in SWR/J mice. Saudi Journal of Biological Sciences. 2022;**29**(3):1543-1549

[84] Zeng J-Y et al. Bisphenol a analogues in associations with serum hormone levels among reproductive-aged Chinese men. Environment International. 2022;**167**:107446

[85] Krzastek SC et al. Impact of environmental toxin exposure

on male fertility potential. Translational Andrology and Urology. 2020;**9**(6):2797-2813

[86] Chianese R et al. Bisphenol a in reproduction: Epigenetic effects. Current Medicinal Chemistry. 2018;**25**(6):748-770

[87] Chen Z et al. Long-term exposure to a 'safe' dose of bisphenol a reduced protein acetylation in adult rat testes. Scientific Reports. 2017;7:40337

[88] Ryu D-Y et al. Abnormal histone replacement following BPA exposure affects spermatogenesis and fertility sequentially. Environment International. 2022;**170**:107617

[89] González-Rojo S et al. Male exposure to bisphenol a impairs spermatogenesis and triggers histone hyperacetylation in zebrafish testes. Environmental Pollution (Barking, Essex: 1987). 2019;**248**:368-379

[90] Chen P-P et al. Associations between urinary bisphenol a and its analogues and semen quality: A cross-sectional study among Chinese men from an infertility clinic. Environment International. 2022;**161**:107132

[91] Jian J-M et al. Global distribution of perfluorochemicals (PFCs) in potential human exposure source-a review. Environment International. 2017;**108**:51-62

[92] Fenton SE et al. Per- and Polyfluoroalkyl substance toxicity and human health review: Current state of knowledge and strategies for informing future research. Environmental Toxicology and Chemistry. 2021;**40**(3):606-630

[93] Joensen UN et al. Do perfluoroalkyl compounds impair human semen quality? Environmental Health Perspectives. 2009;**117**(6):923-927

[94] Schiff JD, Ramírez ML, Bar-Chama N. Medical and surgical management male infertility. Endocrinology and Metabolism Clinics of North America. 2007;**36**(2):313-331

[95] Holm M et al. Leydig cell micronodules are a common finding in testicular biopsies from men with impaired spermatogenesis and are associated with decreased testosterone/LH ratio. The Journal of Pathology. 2003;**199**(3):378-386

[96] Lu T et al. Putative adverse outcome pathways of the male reproductive toxicity derived from toxicological studies of perfluoroalkyl acids. The Science of the Total Environment. 2023;**873**:162439

[97] Liu W, Zeng M, Fu N. Functions of nuclear receptors SUMOylation. Clinica Chimica Acta; International Journal of Clinical Chemistry. 2021;**516**:27-33

[98] Ryu H-Y, Hochstrasser M. Histone sumoylation and chromatin dynamics. Nucleic Acids Research. 2021;**49**(11):6043-6052

[99] Huang W et al. LncRNA-mediated DNA methylation: An emerging mechanism in cancer and beyond. Journal of Experimental & Clinical Cancer Research: CR. 2022;**41**(1):100

[100] Zoch A et al. SPOCD1 is an essential executor of piRNA-directed de novo DNA methylation. Nature. 2020;**584**(7822):635-639

[101] Nilsson EE, Skinner MK. Environmentally induced epigenetic transgenerational inheritance of reproductive disease. Biology of Reproduction. 2015;**93**(6):145

Chapter 3

Fetal Origin Programming of the Male Reproductive System

Yasuko Fujisawa and Ogata Tsutomu

Abstract

The Developmental Origin of Health and Disease (DOHaD) theory, in which the prenatal environment is involved in the development of diseases after birth, has been widely accepted. This theory is widely accepted, and the involvement of the prenatal environment in the development of adult diseases (lifestyle diseases) is almost certain. As an extension of the DOHaD theory, the Testicular Dysgenesis Syndrome (TDS) hypothesis, which focuses specifically on diseases of the male reproductive system, proposes that environmental changes during the embryonic period are involved in the development of a number of diseases of the male reproductive system, such as hypospadias, cryptorchidism, low sperm count, and infertility. A few experimental studies were performed; however, the results have been limited and have not addressed the pathogenic mechanism of TDS. We have conducted research using a mouse model of maternal nutritional deprivation. In this study, under/hyponutrition during fetal life impairs testosterone production in the fetal testis and causes a decrease in sperm count after growth. Further studies elucidated that this may be due to oxidative stress-induced germ cell apoptosis caused by fetal testosterone depletion. The molecular biological background to the DOHaD theory is epigenetic modification, but very few studies have focused on epigenetic modification in TDS, which shares the same background as the DOHaD phenomenon. We will further discuss the contribution of epigenomic modifications in the development of TDS.

Keywords: developmental origin of health and diseases, testicular dysgenesis syndrome, maternal under/hyponutrition, male infertility, epigenomic modification

1. Introduction

The Developmental Origin of Health and Disease (DOHaD) theory that posits the prenatal environment is involved in the development of diseases after birth is widely accepted, and the involvement of the prenatal environment in the development of adult diseases has been established [1]. Furthermore, as an extension of the DOHaD theory, the Testicular Dysgenesis Syndrome (TDS) hypothesis, which particularly focuses on male reproductive system diseases, has been proposed by Professor Skakkebeak in Denmark [2, 3]. This hypothesis proposes that environmental changes during the embryonic period are involved in the development of a series of male reproductive system diseases, such as hypospadias, cryptorchidism, testicular cancer, decreased sperm count, and infertility. The pathogenesis of TDS is assumed to be reduced male hormone (testosterone) action due to testicular damage during the embryonic period [4].

2. Fetal growth restriction (FGR) and male reproductive system disorder

Nutrition and metabolism are essential factors when discussing the prenatal environment. Maternal undernutrition is one of the important causes of FGR [5]. It has been reported that FGR is strongly associated with mild phenotype disorder of sex development/differentiation including hypospadias [6, 7] and cryptorchidism [8–10]. Furthermore, a recent, large cohort study on the relationship between birth records and fertility has been reported from Denmark [11]. The study included more than 10,000 individuals born between 1984 and 1987, consisting of 5342 women and 5342 men. Of these, approximately 10% were born small for gestational age (SGA- a birth weight below the 10th percentile). This study found that there was a 55% increased risk for infertility in men born SGA compared with men born appropriate for gestational age (AGA), not in women. The following study from Sweden also showed that men born SGA or with low birth weight had a lower chance of becoming fathers than men born AGA or with normal birth weight [12]. In addition, an association between FGR and the development of TDS, which considers multiple male reproductive system diseases as a syndrome related to the fetal environment, has been reported by a human study [13]. Together, many epidemiological data from human studies have reported the significant relationship between FGR and wide-ranging male reproductive problems.

Here are several previous reports from basic studies using experimental animals. Maternal 50% food restriction during both gestation and lactation or lactation alone significantly reduced testicular growth in offspring, and also reduced circulating levels of FSH in rats [14]. In an experiment in which pregnant ewes were fed with 50% calory intake in early and late gestation, male lambs born from nutritionally restricted mothers showed a decrease in Sertoli cells in the testis at 10 months of age. Correspondingly, an excess response of FSH in the GnRH loading test was observed [15]. A study in piglets found that maternal calorie restriction during pregnancy reduced Sertoli cells, embryonic cells, and Leydig cells in male piglets born. Apoptotic cells were also found to be more in male piglets from calorie-restricted mothers [16]. Transcriptome analysis in the testes of male pigs revealed that maternal calorie restriction altered a group of genes involved in lipid metabolism, apoptosis, and cell proliferation. In rat offspring, maternal protein restriction during pregnancy reduces the testicular and epidydimal sperm count and affects fertility in the rat offspring [17–19].

Although these experiments provide scientific support for the association between maternal nutrition and the development of male reproductive problems after birth, basic data are still scarce, and the molecular biological background is in the process of being elucidated.

3. Importance of energy metabolism in various aspects of the testis

The testis is the organ responsible for spermatogenesis and the secretion of the major male hormone testosterone. Energy metabolism in the testis has been shown to be important for differentiation and development of testis, and maintenance of testicular function.

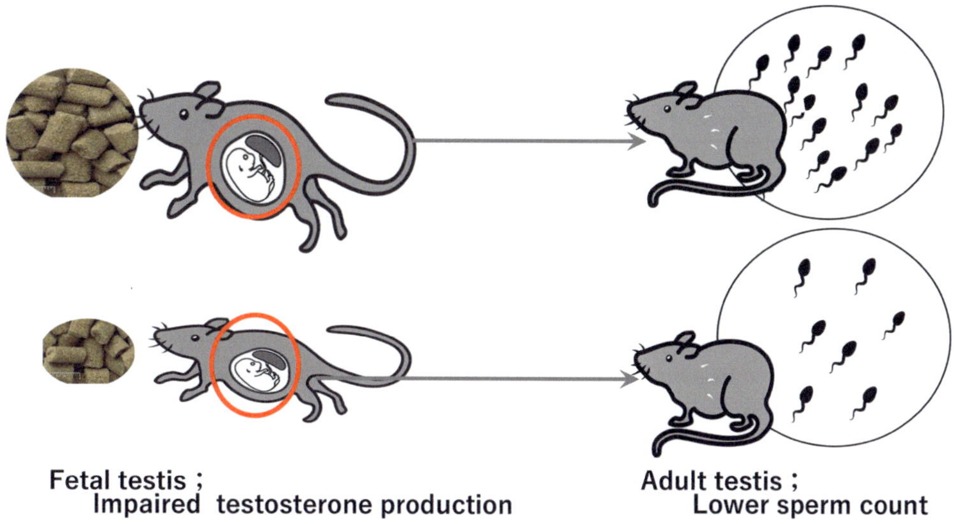

Figure 1.
Maternal caloric restriction resulted in decreased sperm counts after birth (Fujisawa et al. [24]).

In mice, a key event in the early stages of testis differentiation is the activation of Sex-determining region Y (SRY) in pre-Sertoli cells in the gonadal ridges. At this time, testis-specific glycogen accumulates in the pre-sertoli cells. This serves to store an energy source for morphogenesis and hormone production during testis development [20]. Sertoli cell differentiation, a central event in testis formation, requires SRY expression and subsequent SRY-Box9 (SOX9) activation. Through glucose deprivation and metabolic rescue experiments in mice genital ridge cultures, it was demonstrated that an adequate supply of glucose was the most important environment for establishing SOX9 activation in testis differentiation [21]. Additionally, during the differentiation of fetal Leydig cells in mice, a number of genes involved in metabolic pathways, such as tricarboxylic acid cycle, glycolysis, and oxidative phosphorylation, are heavily expressed [22]. Turning to germ cells primordial germ cells (PGCs), the origin of germ cells are found to have very different energy metabolism from pluripotent stem cells (PSCs). Furthermore, for the differentiation of PSCs into PGCs, oxidative phosphorylation is essential [23]. Together, the unique energy metabolic system is important for establishing and maintaining PGC characteristics.

These results suggest that proper nutrition and metabolism play a crucial role in the growth and functioning of the testes. Therefore, it has been hypothesized that intrauterine malnutrition contributes to the emergence of "testicular dysgenesis syndrome (TDS)," which is primarily brought on by unfavorable environmental factors during fetal life and is linked to a number of reproductive abnormalities, such as hypospadias, cryptorchidism, and infertility (**Figure 1**).

4. Intrauterine under/hyponutrition leads to male reproductive dysfunction

Previous studies have shown that maternal under/hyponutrition is thought to increase the chance of developing TDS in the human. However, the underlying mechanism(s) remain largely unknown despite some experimental studies. To clarify

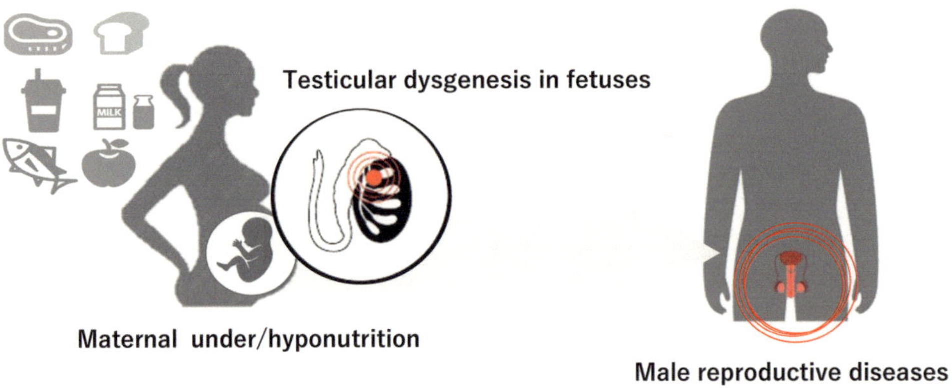

Figure 2.
Maternal under/hyponutrition and male reproductive diseases associated with testicular dysgenesis in fetuses.

the underlying mechanism(s), we performed experimental studies using mice. We set two groups: control females (C-females) were given regular food ad libitum throughout the course of pregnancy while calorie-restricted females (R-females) received 50% of the C-females' mean daily intake from 6.5 dpc. Then, we evaluated male reproductive results between 17.5-days post-coitum-old male mice delivered from C-females (C-fetuses) and those from R-females (R-fetuses) and between six-week-old male mice born to C-females (C-offspring) and those born to R-females (R-offspring) (**Figure 2**) [24].

The external genitalia of the R-fetuses were morphologically normal. However, the anogenital distance (AGD) index (AGDI) calculated by dividing the AGD by the cube root of body weight was significantly shorter in the male R-fetuses than in the male C-fetuses. This indicates reduced exposure to androgen during the fetal period. Intratesticular testosterone levels were significantly low in the R-fetuses compared with the C-fetuses, in association with significantly reduced expressions of steroidogenic genes including *Star, Cyp11a1, Cyp17a1, Hsd3b1, and Hsd17b3.* In contrast, the testicular histopathological findings were comparable between C-fetuses and R-fetuses. Altogether, it is inferred that intrauterine under/hyponutrition compromises fetal testosterone production primarily via the hypofunction of fetal steroidogenic cells. Further, *Nr5a1* (also known as *Sf-1* and *Ad4bp*) and *Insl3* expression levels were considerably lower in R-fetuses than in C-fetuses. The master gene known as *Nr5a1* has been shown to up-regulate the expression of steroidogenic genes as well as *Insl3* [25]. Interestingly, in addition to controlling INSL3 expression, NR5A1 also regulates the intracellular ATP and NADPH concentrations necessary for *de novo* steroid biosynthesis from acetyl-CoA [26, 27] and the generation of *de novo* cholesterol from acetyl-CoA [25]. Thus, compromised *Nr5a1* gene expression might have played an important role in the development of reduced testosterone production in the fetal testis. On the other hand, *Sox9* and *Amh* expressions were similar between the C-fetuses and the R-fetuses despite their expressions being up-regulated by *Nr5a1* [28]. We speculate that *Sox9* and *Amh* expressions are controlled by multiple genes, in cooperation with *Nr5a1* [29, 30].

Furthermore, sperm count was significantly lower in the R-offspring than in the C-offspring at 6 weeks of age while the testicular size and sperm motility were comparable between the two groups. In addition, the number of the R-offspring's TUNEL-positive cells—which are apoptotic cells—was noticeably larger than the

C-offspring's. Moreover, the number of tubules containing TUNEL-positive cells was much higher in the R-offspring than in the C-offspring, and the percentage of TUNEL-positive cells per 100 tubules was obviously high in the R-offspring. The examined sperms must have been generated during the perinatal period, when it is expected that the intratesticular testosterone in R-fetuses is still low, taking into consideration the length of spermatogenesis and movement from the testis to the cauda epididymis [31]. Given that it has been reported that testosterone deprivation leads to germ cell apoptosis [32], a low testosterone environment during the fetal period is likely to be associated with lower sperm count induced by cell apoptosis.

Microarray analysis on the testis in offspring at 6 weeks of age revealed more than 1000 genes that showed significant variation. Next, we picked two genes that showed up-regulation and eight genes that showed down-regulation that were reportedly important for spermatogenic activity. The R-offspring showed considerably up-regulated expressions of *Notch1* and *Esr2* and considerably down-regulated expressions of *Amhr2, Dazl, Hormad1, Nr0b1* (also known as *Dax1*), *Gja1*, *Stra8*, and *Inha*, according to RT-qPCR. *Notch1* and *Esr2* were shown to be up-regulated, and it has been reported that *Notch1* gain-of-function in germ cells causes spermatogenic failure in mice [33] and activation of *Esr2* causes spermatocyte apoptosis and spermiation failure [34]. *Amhr2*, *Dazl*, *Hormad1*, *Nr0b1*, *Gja1*, *Stra8*, and *Inha* were revealed to be down-regulated. According to reports, *AMHR2* is expressed in Sertoli cells as well as spermatocytes, and in humans, *AMHR2* mutations are frequently linked to infertility [35, 36]; spermatogenic failure is linked to *DAZL* polymorphisms in humans, and male *DAZL* knockout (KO) animals exhibit spermatogenic failure [37, 38]; *Hormad1* contributes to the production of synaptonemal complexes, and male and female mice with the *Hormad1* KO mutation are infertile [39]; male *Nr0b1* KO mice exhibit progressive spermatogenic failure and subsequent infertility, and *Nr0b1* is essential for the development of the adrenal and reproductive systems [40, 41]; sertoli cells and germ cells are connected by the testicular gap junction protein *Gja1*, and *Gja1* knockout male mice are infertile as a result of maturation arrest [42, 43]; *Stra8* is solely expressed in germ cells, and *Stra8* KO mice, both male and female, are unable to commence meiosis [44]; and male mice with *Inha* heterozygous KO have decreased spermatogenic activity and *Inha* is significantly expressed in Sertoli cells [45, 46]. Altogether, maternal under/hyponutrition is likely to alter expressions of multiple genes, which could exert an accumulative deleterious effect on spermatogenesis.

Of note, by microarray analysis at 6 weeks of age, the R-offspring showed lower expressions of *Gstp1, Gpx1, Prdx1,* and *Prdx2* [32, 47–50] with anti-oxidative stress and elevated expression of *Nox4* mediating oxidative stress. While anti-apoptotic *Bcl2l1* was upregulated and pro-apoptotic *Bax* and *Bid* and apoptosis-related protease *Casp6* were down-regulated [51–53], this may be explained as the protective responses against the occurrence of apoptosis, probably induced by enhanced oxidative stress. The findings, along with the earlier data, such as the link between low testosterone and oxidative stress-induced apoptosis activation, indicate that TDS is an element of the clinical spectrum of DOHAD and that decreased fetal testosterone production is the main underlying cause of TDS development in intrauterine under/hyponutrition.

5. Epigenomic modifications as the biological basis for the TDS hypothesis

TDS can be considered part of the clinical spectrums of DOHaD theory. This theory proposes that epigenetic changes occurring during fetal and early neonatal period determine disease risk and health [51]. In fact, a number of epigenetic changes have been reported to occur during early life induced by nutritional conditions [52]. Thus, the pathophysiological background of TDS would contain epigenomic modification. Very few studies have focused on epigenomic modifications in TDS, which shares a common background with the DOHaD phenomenon. Recently the epigenome during gametogenesis is altered by factors such as nutritional environment and aging, and can cause multiple diseases.

For example, DNA methylation in sperm due to aging increases or decreases in specific genomic regions [53, 54]. Furthermore, the histone modification H3K4me3 in sperm acts as an apologetic sensor for folate deficiency and obesity [55] and H3K9me2 in spermatozoa is reduced by protein deficiency in [56]. Together, germline-specific epigenomic regulation mechanisms very likely link to metabolic status. Namely the "metabolic-epigenomic crosstalk", in which intracellular metabolic changes lead to epigenomic changes, may function during gametogenesis. Furthermore, non-coding RNAs (ncRNAs), which regulate gene expressions and chromatin structure has been found to involve in the epigenetic program. Recently, environmental stressors such as environmental chemicals have been shown to induce TDS-like symptoms in the next generation through ncRNA-mediated epigenetic modifications in the germline of pups [57, 58]. These findings suggest that research focusing on the importance of epigenomic modification mechanisms as a pathogenic mechanism of TDS is expected to be developed in near future.

Author details

Yasuko Fujisawa* and Ogata Tsutomu
Hamamatsu University School of Medicine, Pediatrics, Hamamatsu, Shizuoka, Japan

*Address all correspondence to: yasuko@hama-med.ac.jp

References

[1] Gluckman PD, Hanson MA. Living with the past: Evolution, development, and patterns of disease. Science. 2004;**305**(5691):1733-1736. DOI: 10.1126/science.1095292

[2] Skakkebaek NE. Testicular dysgenesis syndrome. Hormone Research. 2003;**60**(Suppl. 3):49. DOI: 10.1159/000074499

[3] Sharpe RM, Skakkebaek NE. Testicular dysgenesis syndrome: Mechanistic insights and potential new downstream effects. Fertility and Sterility. 2008;**89**(2 Suppl):e33-e38. DOI: 10.1016/j.fertnstert.2007.12.026

[4] Joensen UN, Jorgensen N, Rajpert-De Meyts E, Skakkebaek NE. Testicular dysgenesis syndrome and Leydig cell function. Basic and Clinical Pharmacology and Toxicology. 2008;**102**(2):155-161. DOI: 10.1111/j.1742-7843.2007.00197.x

[5] Belkacemi L, Nelson DM, Desai M, Ross MG. Maternal undernutrition influences placental-fetal development. Biology of Reproduction. 2010;**83**(3):325-331. DOI: 10.1095/biolreprod.110.084517

[6] Nordenvall AS, Frisen L, Nordenstrom A, Lichtenstein P, Nordenskjold A. Population based nationwide study of hypospadias in Sweden, 1973 to 2009: Incidence and risk factors. Journal of Urology. 2014;**191**(3):783-789. DOI: 10.1016/j.juro.2013.09.058

[7] Gatti JM, Kirsch AJ, Troyer WA, Perez-Brayfield MR, Smith EA, Scherz HC. Increased incidence of hypospadias in small-for-gestational age infants in a neonatal intensive-care unit. BJU International. 2001;**87**(6):548-550

[8] Jensen HI, Ammentorp J, Erlandsen M, Ording H. End-of-life practices in Danish ICUs: Development and validation of a questionnaire. BMC Anesthesiology. 2012;**12**:16. DOI: 10.1016/j.pedneo.2020.07.011

[9] Nemec SF, Nemec U, Brugger PC, Bettelheim D, Weber M, Graham JM Jr, et al. Male genital abnormalities in intrauterine growth restriction. Prenatal Diagnosis. 2012;**32**(5):427-431. DOI: 10.1002/pd.3831

[10] Barthold JS. Undescended testis: Current theories of etiology. Current Opinion in Urology. 2008;**18**(4):395-400. DOI: 10.1002/pd.3831

[11] Thorsted A, Lauridsen J, Hoyer B, Arendt LH, Bech B, Toft G, et al. Birth weight for gestational age and the risk of infertility: A Danish cohort study. Human Reproduction. 2020;**35**(1):195-202. DOI: 10.1093/humrep/dez232

[12] Liffner S, Bladh M, Nedstrand E, Hammar M, Martinez HR, Sydsjo G. Men born small for gestational age or with low birth weight do not improve their rate of reproduction over time: A Swedish population-based study. Fertility and Sterility. 2021;**116**(3):721-730. DOI: 10.1016/j.fertnstert.2021.05.078

[13] Xing JS, Bai ZM. Is testicular dysgenesis syndrome a genetic, endocrine, or environmental disease, or an unexplained reproductive disorder? Life Sciences. 2018;**194**:120-129. DOI: 10.1016/j.lfs.2017.11.039

[14] Leonhardt M, Lesage J, Croix D, Dutriez-Casteloot I, Beauvillain JC, Dupouy JP. Effects of perinatal maternal food restriction on pituitary-gonadal axis and plasma leptin level in rat pup

at birth and weaning and on timing of puberty. Biolpgy of Reproduction. 2003;**68**(2):390-400. DOI: 10.1095/biolreprod.102.003269

[15] Kotsampasi B, Balaskas C, Papadomichelakis G, Chadio SE. Reduced Sertoli cell number and altered pituitary responsiveness in male lambs undernourished in utero. Animal Reproductive Science. 2009;**114**(1-3):135-147. DOI: 10.1016/j.anireprosci.2008.08.017

[16] Lin Y, Xu XY, Wu D, Lin H, Fang ZF, Feng B, et al. Maternal energy insufficiency affects testicular development of the offspring in a swine model. Scientific Reports. 2019;**9**(1):14533. DOI: 10.1016/j.anireprosci.2008.08.017

[17] Toledo FC, Perobelli JE, Pedrosa FP, Anselmo-Franci JA, Kempinas WD. In utero protein restriction causes growth delay and alters sperm parameters in adult male rats. Reproductive Bioligt and Endocrinology. 2011;**9**:94. DOI: 10.1186/1477-7827-9-94

[18] Zambrano E, Bautista CJ, Deas M, Martinez-Samayoa PM, Gonzalez-Zamorano M, Ledesma H, et al. A low maternal protein diet during pregnancy and lactation has sex- and window of exposure-specific effects on offspring growth and food intake, glucose metabolism and serum leptin in the rat. Journal of Physiology. 2006;**571**(Pt 1):221-230. DOI: 10.1113/jphysiol.2005.100313

[19] Zambrano E, Rodriguez-Gonzalez GL, Guzman C, Garcia-Becerra R, Boeck L, Diaz L, et al. A maternal low protein diet during pregnancy and lactation in the rat impairs male reproductive development. Journal of Physiology. 2005;**563**(Pt 1):275-284. DOI: 10.1113/jphysiol.2004.078543

[20] Matoba S, Kanai Y, Kidokoro T, Kanai-Azuma M, Kawakami H, Hayashi Y, et al. A novel Sry-downstream cellular event which preserves the readily available energy source of glycogen in mouse sex differentiation. Journal of Cell Sciences. 2005;**118**(Pt 7):1449-1459. DOI: 10.1242/jcs.01738

[21] Matoba S, Hiramatsu R, Kanai-Azuma M, Tsunekawa N, Harikae K, Kawakami H, et al. Establishment of testis-specific SOX9 activation requires high-glucose metabolism in mouse sex differentiation. Developmental Biology. 2008;**324**(1):76-87. DOI: 10.1016/j.ydbio.2008.09.004

[22] Inoue M, Shima Y, Miyabayashi K, Tokunaga K, Sato T, Baba T, et al. Isolation and characterization of fFetal Leydig progenitor cells of male mice. Endocrinology. 2016;**157**(3):1222-1233. DOI: 10.1210/en.2015-1773

[23] Hayashi Y, Otsuka K, Ebina M, Igarashi K, Takehara A, Matsumoto M, et al. Distinct requirements for energy metabolism in mouse primordial germ cells and their reprogramming to embryonic germ cells. Proceedings of the National Academy of Sciences of the United States of America. 2017;**114**(31):8289-8294. DOI: 10.1073/pnas.1620915114

[24] Fujisawa Y, Ono H, Konno A, Yao I, Itoh H, Baba T, et al. Intrauterine hyponutrition reduces fetal testosterone production and postnatal sperm count in the mouse. Journal of Endocrogy Society. 2022;**6**(4):bvac022. DOI: 10.1210/jendso/bvac022

[25] Lin L, Achermann JC. Steroidogenic factor-1 (SF-1, Ad4BP, NR5A1) and disorders of testis development. Sexual Development. 2008;**2**(4-5):200-209. DOI: 10.1159/000152036

[26] Baba T, Otake H, Inoue M, Sato T, Ishihara Y, Moon JY, et al. Ad4BP/SF-1

regulates cholesterol synthesis to boost the production of steroids. Communications Biology. 2018;**1**:18. DOI: 10.1038/s42003-018-0020-z

[27] Baba T, Otake H, Sato T, Miyabayashi K, Shishido Y, Wang CY, et al. Glycolytic genes are targets of the nuclear receptor Ad4BP/SF-1. Nature Communiations. 2014;**5**:3634. DOI: 10.1038/ncomms4634

[28] Li B, Baba T, Miyabayashi K, Sato T, Shima Y, Ichinose T, et al. Role of Ad4-binding protein/steroidogenic factor 1 in regulating NADPH production in adrenocortical Y-1 cells. Endocrine Journal. 2017;**64**(3):315-324. DOI: 10.1507/endocrj.EJ16-0467

[29] Vining B, Ming Z, Bagheri-Fam S, Harley V. Diverse regulation but conserved function: SOX9 in vertebrate sex determination. Genes (Basel). 2021;**12**(4):486, 1-23. DOI: 10.3390/genes12040486

[30] Teixeira J, Maheswaran S, Donahoe PK. Mullerian inhibiting substance: An instructive developmental hormone with diagnostic and possible therapeutic applications. Endocrine Reveiws. 2001;**22**(5):657-674. DOI: 10.1210/edrv.22.5.0445

[31] McCarrey JR. Toward a more precise and informative nomenclature describing fetal and neonatal male germ cells in rodents. Biology of Reproduction. 2013;**89**(2):47. DOI: 10.1095/biolreprod.113.110502

[32] Kuroda J, Ago T, Matsushima S, Zhai P, Schneider MD, Sadoshima J. NADPH oxidase 4 (Nox4) is a major source of oxidative stress in the failing heart. Proceedings of the National Academy of Sciences of the United States of America. 2010;**107**(35):15565-15570. DOI: 10.1073/pnas.1002178107

[33] Huang Z, Rivas B, Agoulnik AI. NOTCH1 gain of function in germ cells causes failure of spermatogenesis in male mice. PLoS One. 2013;**8**(7):e71213. DOI: 10.1371/journal.pone.0071213

[34] Dumasia K, Kumar A, Deshpande S, Sonawane S, Balasinor NH. Differential roles of estrogen receptors, ESR1 and ESR2, in adult rat spermatogenesis. Molecular and Cellular Endocrinology. 2016;**428**:89-100. DOI: 10.1016/j.mce.2016.03.024

[35] Ohyama K, Ohta M, Hosaka YZ, Tanabe Y, Ohyama T, Yamano Y. Expression of anti-Mullerian hormone and its type II receptor in germ cells of maturing rat testis. Endocrine Journal. 2015;**62**(11):997-1006. DOI: 10.1507/endocrj.EJ15-0370

[36] Mullen RD, Ontiveros AE, Moses MM, Behringer RR. AMH and AMHR2 mutations: A spectrum of reproductive phenotypes across vertebrate species. Developmental Biology. 2019;**455**(1):1-9. DOI: 10.1016/j.ydbio.2019.07.006

[37] Teng YN, Lin YM, Lin YH, Tsao SY, Hsu CC, Lin SJ, et al. Association of a single-nucleotide polymorphism of the deleted-in-azoospermia-like gene with susceptibility to spermatogenic failure. Journal of Clinical Endocrinol Metab. 2002;**87**(11):5258-5264. DOI: 10.1210/jc.2002-020016

[38] Schrans-Stassen BH, Saunders PT, Cooke HJ, de Rooij DG. Nature of the spermatogenic arrest in Dazl −/− mice. Biology of Reproduction. 2001;**65**(3):771-776. DOI: 10.1095/biolreprod65.3.771

[39] Daniel K, Lange J, Hached K, Fu J, Anastassiadis K, Roig I, et al. Meiotic homologue alignment and its quality surveillance are controlled by mouse

HORMAD1. Nature Cell Biology. 2011;**13**(5):599-610. DOI: 10.1038/ncb2213

[40] Lalli E, Sassone-Corsi P. DAX-1, an unusual orphan receptor at the crossroads of steroidogenic function and sexual differentiation. Molecular Endocrinology. 2003;**17**(8):1445-1453. DOI: 10.1210/me.2003-0159

[41] Yu RN, Ito M, Saunders TL, Camper SA, Jameson JL. Role of Ahch in gonadal development and gametogenesis. Nature Genetics. 1998;**20**(4):353-357. DOI: 10.1038/3822

[42] Pointis G, Fiorini C, Defamie N, Segretain D. Gap junctional communication in the male reproductive system. Biochimica et Biophysica Acta. 2005;**1719**(1-2):102-116. DOI: 10.1016/j.bbamem.2005.09.017

[43] Roscoe WA, Barr KJ, Mhawi AA, Pomerantz DK, Kidder GM. Failure of spermatogenesis in mice lacking connexin43. Biology of Reproduction. 2001;**65**(3):829-838. DOI: 10.1095/biolreprod65.3.829

[44] Anderson EL, Baltus AE, Roepers-Gajadien HL, Hassold TJ, de Rooij DG, van Pelt AM, et al. Stra8 and its inducer, retinoic acid, regulate meiotic initiation in both spermatogenesis and oogenesis in mice. Proceedings of the National Academy of Sciences of the United States of America. 2008;**105**(39):14976-14980. DOI: 10.1073/pnas.0807297105

[45] Barakat B, O'Connor AE, Gold E, de Kretser DM, Loveland KL. Inhibin, activin, follistatin and FSH serum levels and testicular production are highly modulated during the first spermatogenic wave in mice. Reproduction. 2008;**136**(3):345-359. DOI: 10.1530/REP-08-0140

[46] Itman C, Bielanowicz A, Goh H, Lee Q, Fulcher AJ, Moody SC, et al. Murine inhibin alpha-subunit Haploinsufficiency causes transient abnormalities in Prepubertal testis development followed by adult testicular decline. Endocrinology. 2015;**156**(6):2254-2268. DOI: 10.1210/en.2014-1555

[47] Sharma R, Yang Y, Sharma A, Awasthi S, Awasthi YC. Antioxidant role of glutathione S-transferases: Protection against oxidant toxicity and regulation of stress-mediated apoptosis. Antioxidants and Redox Signaling. 2004;**6**(2):289-300. DOI: 10.1089/152308604322899350

[48] Lubos E, Loscalzo J, Handy DE. Glutathione peroxidase-1 in health and disease: From molecular mechanisms to therapeutic opportunities. Antioxidants and Redox Signaling. 2011;**15**(7):1957-1997. DOI: 10.1089/ars.2010.3586

[49] Neumann CA, Krause DS, Carman CV, Das S, Dubey DP, Abraham JL, et al. Essential role for the peroxiredoxin Prdx1 in erythrocyte antioxidant defence and tumour suppression. Nature. 2003;**424**(6948): 561-565. DOI: 10.1038/nature01819

[50] Perkins A, Nelson KJ, Parsonage D, Poole LB, Karplus PA. Peroxiredoxins: Guardians against oxidative stress and modulators of peroxide signaling. Trends in Biochemical Sciences. 2015;**40**(8):435-445. DOI: 10.1016/j.tibs.2015.05.001

[51] Godfrey KM, Barker DJ. Fetal nutrition and adult disease. Americal Journal of Clinical Nutrition. 2000; **71**(5 Suppl):1344S-1352S. DOI: 10.1093/ajcn/71.5.1344s

[52] Jimenez-Chillaron JC, Diaz R, Martinez D, Pentinat T, Ramon-Krauel M, Ribo S, et al. The role of nutrition on epigenetic modifications and their implications on health.

Biochimie. 2012;**94**(11):2242-2263. DOI: 10.1016/j.biochi.2012.06.012

[53] Potabattula R, Zacchini F, Ptak GE, Dittrich M, Muller T, El Hajj N, et al. Increasing methylation of sperm rDNA and other repetitive elements in the aging male mammalian germline. Aging Cell. 2020;**19**(8):e13181

[54] Yoshizaki K, Kimura R, Kobayashi H, Oki S, Kikkawa T, Mai L, et al. Paternal age affects offspring via an epigenetic mechanism involving REST/NRSF. EMBO Reports. 2021;**22**(2):e51524. DOI: 10.1016/j.biochi.2012.06.012

[55] Lismer A, Dumeaux V, Lafleur C, Lambrot R, Brind'Amour J, Lorincz MC, et al. Histone H3 lysine 4 trimethylation in sperm is transmitted to the embryo and associated with diet-induced phenotypes in the offspring. Developmental Cell. 2021;**56**(5):671-686. DOI: 10.1016/j.devcel.2021.01.014

[56] Yoshida K, Maekawa T, Ly NH, Fujita SI, Muratani M, Ando M, et al. ATF7-dependent epigenetic changes are required for the intergenerational effect of a paternal low-protein diet. Molecular Cell. 2020;**78**(3):445-458 e446. DOI: 10.1016/j.molcel.2020.02.028

[57] Stenz L, Escoffier J, Rahban R, Nef S, Paoloni-Giacobino A. Testicular dysgenesis syndrome and long-lasting epigenetic silencing of mouse sperm genes involved in the reproductive system after prenatal exposure to DEHP. PLoS One. 2017;**2017**:13. DOI: 10.1371/journal.pone.0170441

[58] Larriba E, Del Mazo J. Role of non-coding RNAs in the transgenerational epigenetic transmission of the effects of reprotoxicants. International Journal of Molecular Sciences. 2016;**17**(4):452, 1-13. DOI: 10.3390/ijms17040452

Chapter 4

Current Progress on the Curative Effects of Cell-Based Therapy for Patients with Non-Obstructive Azoospermia

Ahmed Atwa, Serag Eldin I. Elbehairi, Sayed Bakry, Ahmed B.M. Mehany, Mahmoud Ashry, Hussam Askar and Mohammad Y. Alfaifi

Abstract

Stem cell therapies hold promise for enhancing infertility treatments through improved differentiation and cytokine secretion mechanisms, particularly autologous stem cells known for safety and compatibility. Collaboration and ongoing research are essential for clinical adoption. Additionally, cell-based treatments offer potential solutions for non-obstructive azoospermia NOA, a condition characterized by absent sperm in ejaculate. Traditional therapies have limitations, prompting exploration of spermatogonial stem cells SSCs and induced pluripotent stem cells iPSCs. Animal studies demonstrate successful fertility restoration *via* SSC transplantation, and progress has been made in characterizing human SSCs. However, challenges persist in expanding human SSCs and optimizing iPSC differentiation. Further research is necessary to overcome technical hurdles, ensure safety, and offer a novel NOA treatment option, ultimately restoring fertility.

Keywords: stem cell therapies, azoospermia, mesenchymal stem cells, fertility restoration, SCC transplantation

1. Introduction

Spermatogenesis comprises three key stages. Initially, it involves the growth and maturation of spermatogonia. Next, meiosis (I and II) occurs, leading to the creation of haploid cells. Finally, spermiogenesis ensues, involving various biochemical and morphological changes in round spermatids. These alterations encompass chromatin compaction, acrosome formation, and flagellum assembly and elongation, ultimately yielding mature spermatozoa. Any anomalies in these specialized processes can hinder sperm cell production, resulting in NOA, which is known to exhibit significant genetic diversity. Studies have identified mutations in over 600 genes as contributors to reduced fertility in animal models [1]. Moreover, within the testis, 2274 genes are notably active, with 474 exclusively expressed in this organ. Presently, there are only two standard genetic tests for individuals affected by NOA. These tests involve karyotype analysis to detect sex chromosome abnormalities, particularly Klinefelter syndrome (47 XXY) and various translocations, as well as the investigation of microdeletions in the AZF region. However, these tests yield a diagnosis for only around 20% of the individuals studied, indicating that most affected individuals remain undiagnosed [2].

Most couples, regardless of diagnosis, desire natural conception. However, those with NOA face a unique challenge. Their only option for pregnancy is testicular sperm extraction (TESE) followed by *in vitro* fertilization (IVF) using intracytoplasmic sperm injection ICSI. Success rates are disappointingly low at 30–50%, making the invasive, time-consuming, emotionally distressing, and costly TESE-ICSI process worth avoiding if chances are slim. Physicians should recommend it only when benefits outweigh risks. Without a precise diagnosis, TESE-ICSI might be futile, overlooking quicker options like sperm donation or adoption. Infertile men, relatives, and potential offspring face increased health risks, notably cancer. Genetic diagnosis, providing prognostic value, is crucial for well-informed guidance during TESE and/or endocrine therapy [3, 4].

The World Health Organization (WHO) recognizes male infertility as a major global health issue affecting over 50 million couples. NOA is a condition where sperm are absent in the ejaculate, even after centrifugation and microscopic examination [5]. It affects about 1% of all males and 10% of males with infertility, with a wide range of genetic causes [6].

Azoospermia, the absence of spermatozoa in ejaculates, can be classified into obstructive and non-obstructive NOA forms. Distinguishing between these types is essential as obstructive azoospermia is more favorable, preserving spermatogenesis. Clinical examination, including evaluation of medical history, hormone levels, and physical examination, provides reliable means to differentiate the two types [7]. However, NOA, which accounts for approximately 10% of infertility cases, is characterized by the absence of spermatozoa due to spermatogenic deficiency. Often, azoospermia is associated with irreversible disorders of the testicles related to endocrine, genetic, and inflammatory diseases [8]. Idiopathic NOA, without a known cause, is also possible [9].

Non-obstructive azoospermia is typically characterized by small and flaccid testicles, as determined by palpation and measurement. In all azoospermia cases, measuring hormone levels such as follicle-stimulating hormone (FSH), luteinizing hormone (LH), prolactin, total testosterone, estradiol, and inhibin B is important [10]. In NOA, FSH levels are usually elevated, LH levels are increased or close to normal, and hypogonadism (low total testosterone) is prevalent, indicating a deficiency in Leydig cells obesity may lead to a reduction in testosterone levels and an elevation in serum estradiol levels, primarily as a result of androgen conversion occurring in peripheral tissues [11]. Nevertheless, in obese individuals, decreased testosterone levels could potentially be attributed to adjustments in sex hormone-binding globulin (SHBG) rather than a genuine deficiency in testosterone [7, 12].

Distinguishing obstructive azoospermia from NOA is crucial for treatment choices and the success of sperm extraction surgery. Men with azoospermia need a hormonal assessment, including FSH and total testosterone measurements [13]. NOA causes can be pretesticular (like endocrine issues) or testicular (acquired or congenital), often leading to elevated FSH levels. Common acquired causes include varicocele, orchitis, chemotherapy exposure, or trauma, detected through medical history and examination [14]. Congenital causes involve chromosomal abnormalities and Y chromosome microdeletions, detected *via* karyotyping and PCR [14, 15]. While primary testicular failure is usually irreversible, advancements like testicular sperm extraction offer a 50% sperm retrieval rate, enabling ICSI but requiring genetic screening [16].

Cellular transplantation addresses male infertility, especially NOA, in two ways: regenerative medicine enhances germ cell proliferation and differentiation while exploiting transplanted cells' paracrine and anti-inflammatory effects to treat NOA caused by idiopathic and inflammatory factors.

2. The limitations of current treatment options and the need for the cell-based therapy

From the perspective of regenerative medicine, there are two experimental approaches aimed at restoring fertility in men with NOA. The first method, referred to as the *in vivo* approach, involves the transplantation of SSCs into the seminiferous tubules of infertile individuals. These SSCs serve as precursors to mature spermatids. On the other hand, the second method is based on *in vitro* studies and involves the cultivation and differentiation of various cell types into male germ cells. These cell types include embryonic stem cells [17], iPSCs [18], and MSCs [19, 20].

The upcoming discussion will focus on restoring fertility in men with NOA using the cell sources shown in **Figure 1**.

Stem cells possess the unique ability to self-renew and differentiate into various human tissue cell types. Among these, MSCs have gained prominence in cellular therapy due to their potential. Derived from sources like bone marrow and adipose tissue, MSCs are prized by researchers and clinicians for their versatility, minimal immune reactivity, and active tissue repair capabilities. Compared to other stem cell types, MSCs offer advantages in clinical cell-based therapies, including easy sourcing, immune-suppressive qualities, suitability for autograft and allograft procedures, ethical acceptability, and limited replicative lifespan [22].

3. Overview of cell-based therapy

Cell and tissue-derived products' origin is pivotal in regenerative medicine. To boost widespread adoption, we must produce ample cells with consistent quality and therapeutic effectiveness. This ensures steady therapeutic outcomes for patients [23].

This section examines various cell sources for cell therapy in different pathological conditions. We will also explore the transition from cell suspensions to complex tissue-engineered products. Diverse cell sources, including adult materials from living and deceased donors, fetal materials, and pluripotent stem cell lines, have been extensively researched in cell therapy and regenerative medicine [23, 24]. Humans possess a complex multicellular structure with specialized cell types, all originating from a single zygote. As development progresses, cells diversify and lose their ability to transform into other cell types. This ability is referred to as "cell potency" [25, 26] (**Table 1**).

Adult cell material, obtained directly from patients, can be purified, or amplified in a lab, for example, mesenchymal stem cells or skin epithelial cells. This self-derived method reduces the risk of rejection but complicates manufacturing and supply logistics for large-scale production [27]. These challenges are more pronounced in diseases like

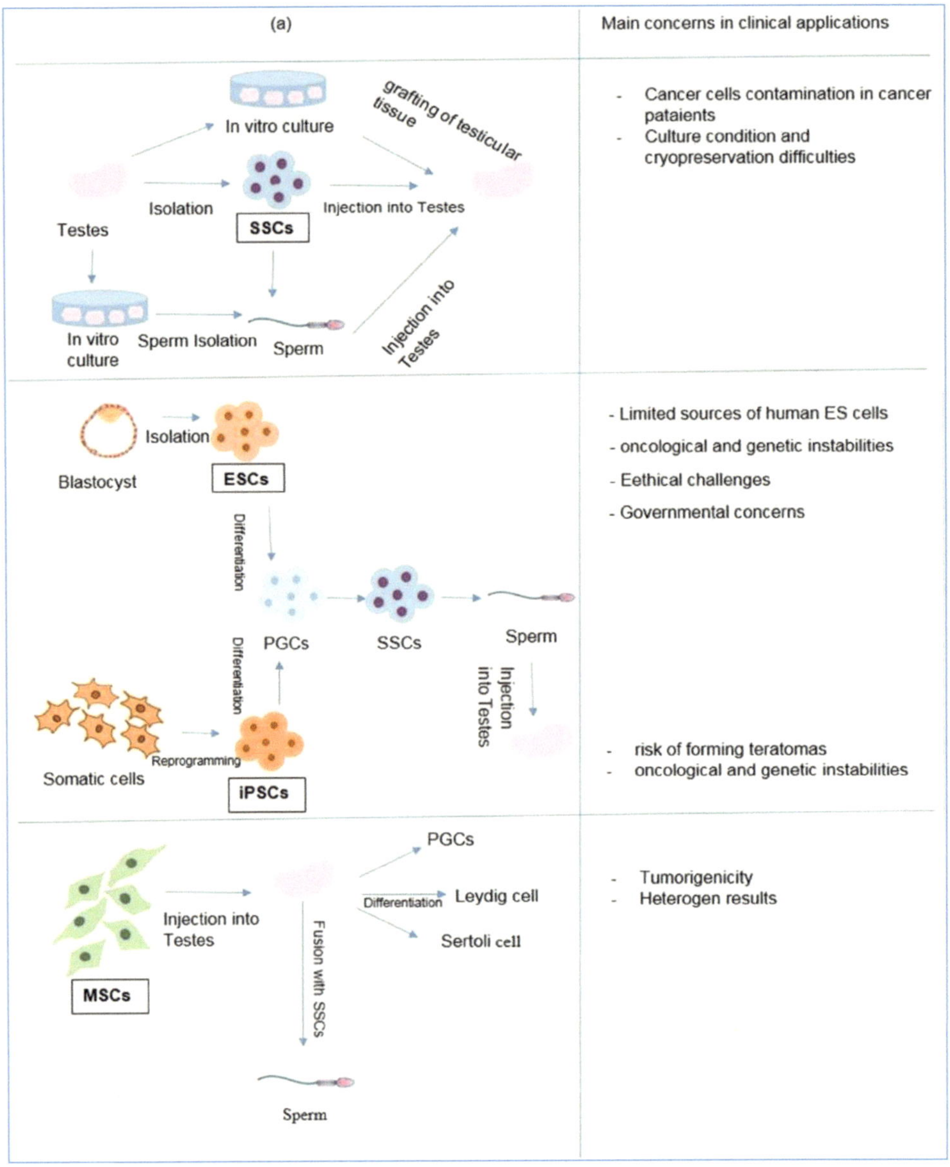

Figure 1.
Cell-based therapy for non-obstructive azoospermia. Regenerative medicine strategies are used for cell-based treatments of NOA. (b) Employing (MSCs and testicular somatic cells (DSCs) in NOA cell-based therapy aims to harness their secreted anti-inflammatory and paracrine factors [21].

age-related macular degeneration (AMD) or when many cells are needed, like extensive burn treatment. Alternatively, cells can come from deceased or, when possible, living donors (see **Figure 2**). Using adult cell sources introduce variability due to donor differences in characteristics like histocompatibility, age, and genotype. Additionally, adult cell sources have limited expansion potential, especially for terminally differentiated types (e.g., skeletal muscle cells) or organs with few endogenous stem cells [29].

Potential sources of materials for cell therapy encompass aborted fetuses, which offer highly proliferative cells compared to adult cells. Fetal stem/progenitor cells

Totipotency	During the blastocyst phase, a solitary cell possesses the capability to generate all cells until the stage of 16 cells.
Pluripotency	Embryonic stem cells can differentiate into cells that belong to all three germ layers.
Multipotency	The activation of genes imposes restrictions on the ability of these cells to differentiate into multiple cell types, albeit within a limited range. For instance, hematopoietic stem cells possess the capability to differentiate into diverse types of blood cells, including erythrocytes, lymphoid cells, neutrophils, and platelets.
Oligopotency	Certain stem cells possess the ability to differentiate into a restricted range of cell types. To illustrate, lymphoid stem cells can undergo development into either B cells or T cells.
Unipotency	Capability to specialize into a solitary cellular form, such as a precursor cell.

Table 1.
Cellular potency.

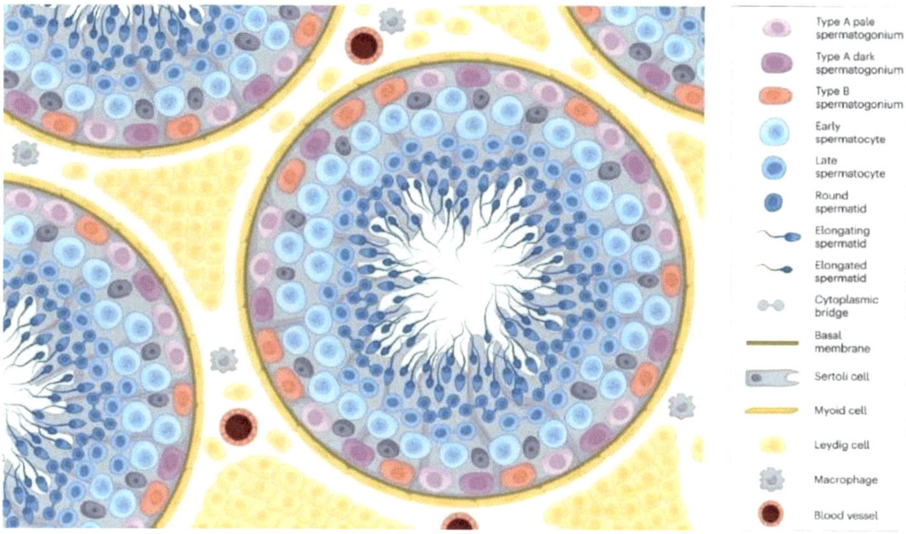

Figure 2.
A simplified diagram showing a cross-section of a seminiferous tubule and the interstitial space around it is presented. The depicted cell-to-cell communication pathways that play a role in spermatogenesis are also indicated. It is important to note that the germ cells are not depicted as isolated entities; instead, they are connected through intercellular bridges, facilitating the exchange of cytoplasmic contents until later stages after meiosis, when these bridges no longer exist [28].

possess limited differentiation potential but can yield cell types absent in adult tissues. The availability of fetal cells varies globally due to diverse abortion laws. Ethical concerns surround the use of human fetal tissue.

Obtaining fetuses at specific gestational stages poses challenges, as seen in the MIG-HD trial for Huntington's disease. They attempted grafting fetal ganglionic eminences (GE), containing potential striatal cells, into HD patients' brains. However, 163 surgeries were canceled out of 86 intended, due to inadequate or substandard fetal material, as fetal cells must be transplanted within 2 days post-abortion [30].

Human pluripotent stem cells hPSCs hold great promise for regenerative medicine due to their remarkable self-renewal and differentiation capabilities. They can be obtained from surplus *in vitro* fertilized embryos, known as human embryonic stem cells hESCs, or by reprogramming adult cells into a pluripotent state, termed human induced pluripotent stem cell hiPSC generation. Large-scale hiPSC production requires strict adherence to quality control standards and good manufacturing practices (GMP), akin to pharmaceuticals. While hESCs have been predominant in clinical trials, the field is increasingly favoring hiPSCs because they eliminate the need to destroy embryos, allowing wider use [31].

Cell therapy involves introducing healthy cells into diseased tissues, utilizing mature cells or undifferentiated stem cells that can adapt to specific conditions (as shown in **Figure 2**). Various treatment categories are available for male infertility, including optimizing sperm production, addressing obstructions, and employing surgical sperm retrieval techniques [32]. Men with NOA often require testicular sperm retrieval methods like testicular sperm extraction (TESA), conventional TESA (cTESE), or microsurgical TESA (micro-TESE). Among these techniques, micro-TESE has demonstrated superior success rates, reduced testicular tissue damage, increased sperm yield, and enhanced potential for sperm cryopreservation compared to alternative methods in NOA cases. Despite these advancements, the clinical pregnancy rate remains disappointingly low [33]. However, there is a glimmer of hope for NOA patients who have experienced unsuccessful pregnancies after undergoing micro-TESE surgery, as stem cell therapy emerges as a potential solution [34].

Mesenchymal stem cell (MSC) transplantation is a novel strategy to stimulate spermatogenesis and address male infertility. Sertoli cells (SCs) are crucial for cell survival, proliferation, migration, angiogenesis, and immune modulation. This makes MSCs an excellent choice for azoospermia treatment [35]. MSCs from bone marrow are a primary MSC source and have demonstrated the ability to differentiate into male germ cells in lab settings [36, 37]. Studies have observed spermatogenesis induction and MSC differentiation into germ cells when transplanted into NOA animal models. BM-MSC allotransplantation has successfully treated azoospermia in various animal models, including guinea pigs [38], hamsters [39], mice [40], and rats [41]. Stem cell therapy has significantly advanced NOA management, as seen in trials like NCT02025270, NCT02641769, and NCT02414295, evaluating bone marrow-derived mesenchymal stem cells (BM-MSCs) effects on hormonal profiles, testicular dimensions, and sexual function in NOA cases.

4. The process of spermatogenesis initiates during puberty, wherein spermatogonia under spermatogonial stem cells: a novel approach for treating impaired spermatogenesis

The process of spermatogenesis begins during puberty, when spermatogonia undergo mitotic and meiotic divisions, resulting in the production of haploid spermatids and spermatozoa. Since spermatogenesis relies heavily on stem cells [42], one potential treatment for male infertility caused by impaired spermatogenesis is the transplantation of stem cells (refer to **Figure 3**). SSCs can restore spermatogenesis in cases where spermatogonial cells have been damaged or depleted [44]. Consequently, stem cell transplantation holds promise as a technique to revive spermatogenesis in cancer patients and individuals experiencing impaired spermatogenesis [45].

Cancer treatments like radiation and chemotherapy can lead to male infertility in cancer patients. Preserving fertility is a major concern for young boys with cancer. To address this, a procedure called testicular biopsy is performed to collect SSCs, which are frozen before cancer treatment. Later, a stem cell transplant is done in the testes. Researchers are also exploring other stem cell types like MSCs, embryonic stem cells

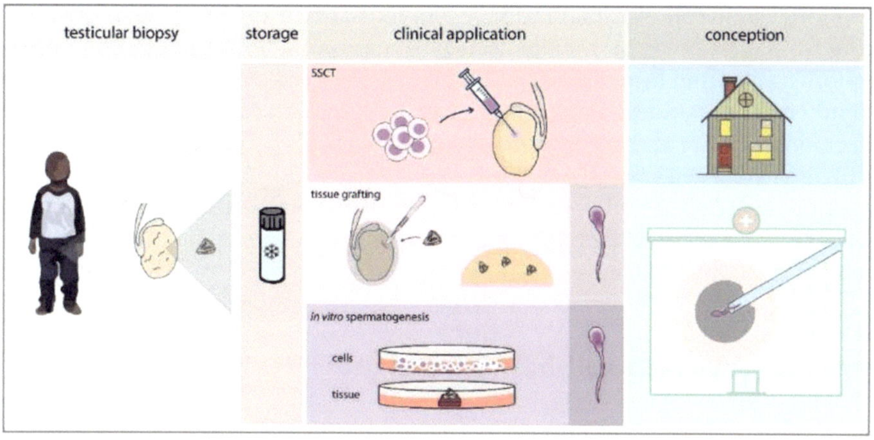

Figure 3.
Fertility restoration routes. Following the freezing of a testicular tissue sample, various methods utilizing SSCs can be employed to restore fertility. These methods include SSC transplantation (SSCT), grafting of testicular tissue, and in vitro spermatogenesis, which can be carried out through either cell-based or tissue-based cultivation. With SSCT, there is potential for natural conception, while techniques involving grafting or in vitro spermatogenesis would require an ICSI procedure using elongated spermatids obtained from the respective method [43].

(ESCs), very small embryonic-like stem cells (VSELs), and iPSCs to tackle azoospermia, which can be derived from regular somatic cells [46, 47].

SSCs possess remarkable self-renewal and pluripotent abilities, as highlighted by Seandel et al. [48]. These cells can differentiate into various stem cell types, playing a pivotal role in spermatogenesis and male fertility. However, SSCs are relatively scarce, comprising only 0.03% of germ cells in rodent testes. In contrast, differentiating cells like spermatogonia, spermatocytes, spermatids, and sperm, as observed by Phillips et al. [49], are more abundant. This balance ensures both stem cell preservation and the high sperm production demands of the testes. The emergence of SSCs presents significant potential for addressing human challenges through biotechnological advancements, as extensively explored in biomedical research, as discussed by Park et al. [50].

SSCs originate from gonocytes within the postnatal testis. These gonocytes trace their lineage back to primordial germ cells (PGCs) that emerge during early embryonic development. PGCs, initially identified as alkaline phosphatase-positive cells in the epiblast-stage embryo, appear around 7–7.25 days post-coitum (dpc) in rodents and around 24 dpc in humans, located near the allantois within the yolk sac wall ("post-coitum" is a widely accepted Latin term in biology and reproductive medicine for events after sexual intercourse) [51]. Human PGC presence relies on BMP4 and BMP8b expression within the extraembryonic ectoderm. PGCs passively migrate from the developing embryo, reaching the forming gonadal ridge between 8.5 and 12.5 dpc in mice and 29 and 33 dpc in humans, with approximately 3000 PGCs populating the genital ridges during this process [52]. Subsequently, PGCs differentiate into gonocytes within the male gonads around 13.5 dpc. These gonocytes are situated within testicular cords, composed of precursor Sertoli and peritubular myoid cells. Gonocytes can be categorized as mitotic (M)-prespermatogonia, T1-prospermatogonia, and T2-prospermatogonia. M prespermatogonia, located centrally within testicular cords, progress through various developmental stages during spermatogenesis [53]. Mitotic and meiotic divisions ultimately yield haploid spermatids and spermatozoa (see **Figure 2**). Given the reliance of spermatogenesis on stem cells, Kanatsu-Shinohara et al. explored stem cell transplantation as a potential solution for male infertility resulting from disrupted spermatogenesis [44], cancer patients undergoing radiation or chemotherapy often face male infertility as a side effect. Preserving fertility is crucial for prepubertal boys undergoing cancer treatment. In such cases, a testicular biopsy is performed to isolate and cryopreserve autologous SSCs before cancer treatment. Subsequently, stem cell transplantation is conducted within the testes, as described by Forbes et al. [46]. Additionally, various other stem cell types, such as MSCs, embryonic stem cells (ESCs), very small embryonic-like stem cells (VSELs), and iPSCs, derived from normal somatic cells, have been explored for treating azoospermia [47].

5. Spermatogonial stem cell-based techniques

The presence of PGCs in humans depends on the expression of BMP4 and BMP8b in the extraembryonic ectoderm [44]. Afterward, PGCs are carried away from the developing embryo during allantois development until they migrate through the hindgut, eventually reaching the developing gonadal ridge. In mice, this migration typically occurs between 8.5 and 12.5 dpc, while in humans, it happens at 29–33 dpc. During this migration, approximately 3000 PGCs colonize the genital ridges. These PGCs eventually give rise to gonocytes, which become enclosed in testicular cords. These cords consist of Sertoli precursor cells and peritubular myoid cells and are present in male gonads at approximately 13.5 dpc. Gonocytes can be further classified into three categories: M-prespermatogonia, T1-prospermatogonia, and T2-prospermatogonia. M-prespermatogonia are located in the middle of the testicular cords, away from the basement membrane, and undergo various developmental stages throughout spermatogenesis [52].

6. *In vitro* proliferation and transplantation of SSCs

The potential restoration of fertility and natural conception in patients through the recolonization of seminiferous tubules and *in vivo* spermatogenesis can be achieved by auto-transplantation of SSCs collected from the patient before treatment (see **Figure 3**). The preferred method for reintroducing SSCs into the human testis is the ultrasonically guided injection of cells in the rete testis, as discussed comprehensively by Gul et al. [54].

Brinster and colleagues have successfully illustrated the establishment of colonization and spermatogenesis within the testes of recipient mice, resulting in offspring possessing the donor haplotype [55]. Additionally, Takashima and Shinohara [56] have reviewed studies demonstrating the accomplishment of SSC auto- or allo-transplantation in diverse mammalian species, encompassing rodents, non-rodents, and non-human primates [57, 58], which has subsequently led to functional spermatogenesis in the recipient organisms.

In human studies, clinical trials involving SSC transplantation have not yet been established. A single report on seven men receiving injections of cryopreserved testicular cells lacks a follow-up report on the outcome of the procedures [59]. However, studies in mice have shown that the number of transplanted SSC colonies gradually decreases during the homing process after transplantation [60], and the success of colonization and donor-derived spermatogenesis within the recipient testis is highly dependent on the concentration of transplanted SSCs [61, 62].

To address limited tissue samples from patients, promoting the expansion of SSCs (spermatogonial stem cells) becomes crucial. This expansion is necessary to generate enough for successful transplantation and re-establishment of seminiferous tubules in the recipient's testicular tissue. Kanatsu-Shinohara and colleagues demonstrated sustained, long-term murine SSC expansion, leading to fertility restoration in sterile recipients [63]. Similarly, long-term propagation of testicular cells has been achieved from both adult sources [64] and pre-pubertal tissues [65]. Human SSCs have been confirmed in humans and validated through xenotransplantation into sterile mice, where they successfully migrated to the niche within seminiferous tubules housing SSCs.

Nevertheless, the task of pinpointing SSCs in testicular tissue or *in vitro* cell cultures remains a formidable challenge. In testicular cell cultures, a mixture of somatic cells and germ cells coexists, with the latter constituting a diverse population of spermatogonia at various stages of differentiation. At present, there is no universally accepted marker that definitively distinguishes human and/or non-human primate SSCs, whether within living organisms or in laboratory cultures. Many frequently employed markers, such as ITGA6, KIT, GPR125, and DAZL, are not exclusive to spermatogonia and are also present in somatic cells within the testicular environment [66, 67]. The expression of other markers, like GFRA1, THY1, and UCHL1, in spermatogonia is also controversial [68, 69]. Moreover, the presence of specific indicators is contingent upon the developmental phase of the testicular tissue [70].

Single-cell sequencing studies have identified different developmental states of germ cells, ranging from State 0 to State 4, each characterized by a unique set of markers, although there may be some overlap [71]. Examples of markers expressed in the earliest state include UTF1 and PIWIL4, with PIWIL4 being more specific [71, 72]. Another potential marker for undifferentiated spermatogonia with SSC characteristics is the LPPR3 protein [73].

Furthermore, it is uncertain whether various types of testicular cells maintain their transcriptomic and metabolic signatures when isolated from their natural niche [67]. The diversity found within testicular cell populations, coupled with the abundance of potential markers at our disposal, poses a challenge when it comes to comparing the outcomes and efficiency of culturing SSCs in different research studies. To advance our comprehension and practical use of SSCs, it is imperative to undertake further investigations geared toward pinpointing specific markers applicable to precisely defined spermatogonial subpopulations. Additionally, functional studies are necessary to assess the *in vitro* SSC potential of these identified markers. When seeking out these markers, it is advisable to prioritize surface markers over nuclear markers, as this approach is likely to be more advantageous for the isolation and enrichment of SSCs from cryopreserved biopsies or post-culture scenarios [43].

Cultural methods and media should support SSC proliferation while preventing their differentiation. In addition to basic nutrients, the culture medium may include specific cytokines, metabolites, hormones, and signaling molecules known to stimulate spermatogonial proliferation. Kanatsu-Shinohara et al. successfully developed a culture protocol in 2003 using StemPro-34 Serum-Free medium for long-term *in vitro* propagation of murine SSCs [63]. Although a similar medium can support long-term propagation of human SSCs [64, 65], the overgrowth of testicular somatic cells in the culture system remains a challenge, as it dilutes the SSC signature over time [63]. Feeder cells are beneficial for the survival of SSCs as they provide mechanical and metabolic support as well as paracrine signals [74, 75]. However, the utilization of external feeder layers is not conducive to clinical implementation. Consequently, somatic cells naturally present in the testicular suspension and facilitating SSC proliferation are employed for SSC cultivation. To prevent excessive proliferation of these somatic cells, the cultivation technique and medium must achieve an optimal equilibrium between the growth of somatic cells and SSCs. Alternatively, testicular somatic cells can be substituted with a synthetic matrix for cellular support, coupled with the supplementation of the medium with nutrients and growth factors to provide the metabolic sustenance typically offered by feeder cells for SSCs. Nonetheless, this process heavily relies on the ability to isolate and separate the somatic cell population from the germ cell population prior to cultivation, a task currently constrained by the absence of a specific SSC marker [76].

Hence, it is imperative to refine the *in vitro* cultivation technique for human SSCs before embarking on clinical applications. Investigating the SSC microenvironment in humans could prove pivotal in the discovery of essential factors essential for the efficient preservation and proliferation of SSCs [77].

7. Experimental models and preclinical studies

Spermatogenesis encompasses a series of physiological, morphological, and biochemical changes that lead to the development of mature sperm cells. However, this process can be disrupted by various factors such as congenital or genetic abnormalities, as well as physical, chemical, and environmental factors. These disruptions can contribute to temporary or permanent infertility [78–80]. According to the latest report from the World Health Organization (WHO), a condition known as azoospermia, which refers to the absence of spermatozoa in the ejaculate, affects approximately 1% of the male population and 10–20% of infertile men [81, 82]. Besides genetic and congenital factors, chemotherapeutic drugs have the potential to substantially disrupt the typical processes of spermatogenesis and sperm characteristics. This disruption can result in the cessation of progenitor cell differentiation and a reduction in the germ cell reservoir [83].

8. Busulfan destroys DNA structure, prevents proliferation and differentiation of SSCs, and initiates apoptosis

Various animal models have been described to induce azoospermia, including busulfan injection [84], testicular heat stress [85], testicular torsion [86], radiation [87], and cryptorchidism induction [88]. Among these, busulfan injection and hyperthermia exposure are two commonly used methods to deplete germ cells from the testes [84, 85].

Busulfan, scientifically referred to as 1,4-butanediol dimethanesulfonate, is commonly utilized for the management of myeloproliferative syndromes, chronic myeloid leukemia (CML), lymphomas, and ovarian cancer [89]. This chemotherapeutic medication decreases the rate at which cells multiply by specifically intervening during the G1 phase of their growth cycle. It accomplishes this by forming connections between DNA proteins or DNA strands, effectively halting cell division during the mitosis/replication phase and instigating apoptosis [84]. Busulfan is also administered to leukemia patients prior to bone marrow transplantation, often in combination with cyclophosphamide and clofarabine, as a myelosuppressive/myeloablative drug [90–92]. However, it is important to note that both short-term and long-term side effects have been reported on various vital organs, including the urinary bladder, liver, skin, gonads, and nervous system [93, 94]. Impaired spermatogenesis has been observed in cancer patients receiving busulfan treatment [95]. The primary objective of this study is to examine the adverse impacts of busulfan on various rat organs, such as the liver, kidneys, testes, and bone marrow, utilizing histological, biochemical, and cytological assessments [41, 89].

The application of Busulfan treatment is intended to reduce germ cells for the purpose of transplantation research. Nevertheless, this method is linked to an inadequate elimination of germ cells, and the challenge of depleting endogenous spermatogenesis is greater in rats when compared to mice employed as recipients [96]. Various research groups have employed different doses (ranging from 10 to 50 mg/kg) of busulfan to eliminate testis function for their experiments, and different mouse strains exhibit varying sensitivities to busulfan doses. Recently, [97] in WBB6F1 WT mice, endogenous resumption was observed at 22 mg/kg busulfan dose, contrasting with the absence of resumption at 44 mg/kg. Our investigation in Swiss mice showed germ cell aplasia at or above 25 mg/kg, with doses exceeding 25 mg/kg causing premature mortality, hindering long-term safety assessment. Therefore, we consistently use a 25 mg/kg dose, achieving superior spermatogenesis restoration after niche cell transplantation compared to vehicle transplants post-chemotherapy. In humans, azoospermia in cancer survivors varies based on specific oncological drugs. A recent study using seven testicular biopsies from adult survivors of childhood cancers found a complete absence of germ cells, with only Sertoli cells and VSELs surviving [98].

9. Effects of heat stress on spermatogenesis and germ cells

Maintaining the temperature of the testicles within an optimal range is crucial for the process of spermatogenesis. Even slight increases in scrotal temperature, even within the normal physiological range, have a detrimental impact on sperm quality [99]. A rise of 1°C results in a 14% reduction in spermatogenesis (see **Figure 4**), leading to decreased sperm production [100]. The influence of temperature on male fertility is evident, as infertile men have higher mean scrotal temperatures compared to fertile men, and further increases in scrotal temperature result in a decline in sperm quality [101].

Spermatogenesis, specifically the process of spermatocyte and spermatid differentiation and maturation, is profoundly influenced by temperature. The ideal conditions for spermatogenesis require a temperature that is at least 2°C lower than the core temperature of the body [102]. However, elevated scrotal temperature leads to testicular germinal atrophy, spermatogenic arrest [103], and reduced levels of inhibin B (a biochemical marker of spermatogenesis) [104], resulting in lower sperm counts [105].

The susceptibility of germ cells to heat stress is higher due to their elevated mitotic activity [106]. Within the germ cell population, pachytene and diplotene spermatocytes, as well as early round spermatids, are particularly susceptible to heat stress in both humans [107] and rats [102, 108]. Several fundamental mechanisms contribute to germ cell damage, including germ cell apoptosis [108], autophagy [109], DNA damage caused by altered synapsis and strand breaks, and the generation of reactive oxygen species. The subsequent section, "Molecular response of male germ cells to heat stress," will provide a more detailed explanation of the molecular reactions observed in germ cells under hyperthermic conditions [85].

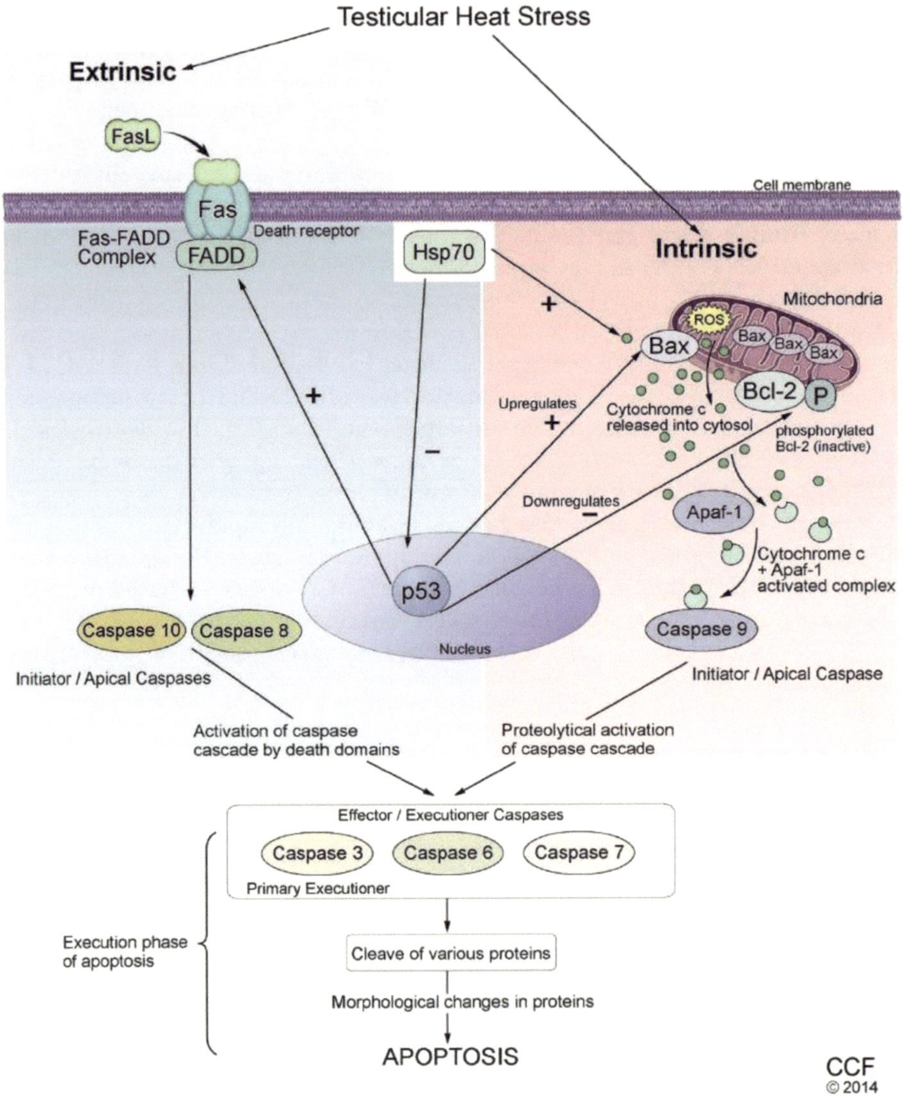

Figure 4.
The pathways involved in apoptosis: intrinsic and extrinsic. The intrinsic pathway centers on mitochondrial regulation, where Bax accumulates in response to heat stress, leading to cytochrome C release and caspase activation. The extrinsic pathway, initiated by Fas-FasL binding, activates caspases via the Fas/FADD complex. In hyperthermia, p53 relocates to the nucleus, inducing cell cycle arrest and apoptosis, while also influencing the intrinsic pathway by regulating Bax and Bcl-2. Both pathways converge at the executioner caspase cascade, resulting in germ cell death [85].

10. Cell-based therapies for NOA *via* paracrine and anti-inflammatory pathways

Scientific evidence suggests that immune-related factors and inflammatory processes could be responsible for testicular damage and male infertility in approximately 30% of asymptomatic infertile patients [110]. Research indicates that immune cell infiltration has been observed in at least 20% of testicular biopsies taken from infertile patients with azoospermia, indicating a significant contribution of inflammatory infertility to male infertility [111].

Prior research has likewise illustrated the existence of immune cell infiltration and simultaneous inflammatory ailments in testicular biopsies from all dogs afflicted with NOA, encompassing M1 pro-inflammatory phenotype macrophages, pro-inflammatory monocytes, and cytokines [112].

In previous research, biopsies collected from males diagnosed with NOA revealed the presence of inflammatory lesions, characterized by the presence of lymphocytes and monocytes/macrophages, which were linked to compromised spermatogenesis. In contrast, samples taken from individuals with obstructive azoospermia (OA) exhibited uninhibited spermatogenesis without any signs of inflammation [113]. These investigations also revealed that inflammatory responses have the potential to inflict harm upon the testes and epididymis. Elevated concentrations of inflammatory mediators like tumor necrosis factor (TNF) and Activin A were detected in human testicular biopsies displaying compromised spermatogenesis, as observed in these studies [114]. Additionally, NOA has been observed in 10% of men with acute epididymitis. As mentioned earlier, (MSCs have been found to possess immunomodulatory, anti-inflammatory, anti-apoptotic, and proliferative effects through the secretion of cytokines and growth factors [115, 116].

Accumulative evidence suggests that the components of the spermatogonial stem cell niche play a significant role in the development of idiopathic male infertility. Infertility affects approximately 8–12% of couples worldwide, with male factors contributing to about 50% of cases. Idiopathic male infertility, accounting for 30–50% of male infertility cases, lacks identifiable causes [117]. Despite normal physical examinations and laboratory tests, semen analysis often reveals sperm abnormalities, either isolated or in combination [118].

Epigenetic elements, specifically alterations in DNA methylation at a global or gene-specific level, could potentially play a role in the onset of idiopathic male infertility. However, the involvement of histone modifications and chromatin protamination in spermatogenesis remains somewhat uncertain [119]. Specific configurations of differential DNA methylation regions may function as prognostic indicators for the efficacy of particular treatments in addressing idiopathic male infertility [120]. Nonetheless, there is a need for more comprehensive research to elucidate the mechanisms responsible for changes in DNA methylation patterns and their significance in the context of male infertility. Likewise, although extensive investigations have been carried out on other epigenetic elements like miRNAs, additional data are essential to establish a definitive link between abnormal miRNA expression and unexplained male infertility [121].

Abnormal mRNA expression could also be correlated with unexplained male infertility. Research has indicated that numerous genes associated with unexplained male infertility are connected to reactive oxygen species (ROS). This might elucidate the observed disproportion in ROS genes and their protein products in seminal plasma and impaired spermatozoa [122]. The expression levels of glutathione transferase genes were discovered to be elevated in samples obtained from individuals afflicted with NOA and oligospermia, which may contribute to the detoxification of reactive oxygen species (ROS) [123]. Aberrant expression is not limited to cells in the spermatogenic epithelium but also extends to somatic cells [124]. Transcriptome analysis of single Sertoli cells obtained from patients with idiopathic male infertility revealed the presence of immature Sertoli cell fractions. These cells exhibited characteristics resembling infantile and pubertal Sertoli cells, displayed increased in vitro proliferation, and demonstrated energy metabolism patterns typical of immature Sertoli cells. Although their ability to support germ cell colonies was slightly impaired compared to normal adult Sertoli cells, this functional immaturity could be reversed through inhibition of the Wnt pathway, suggesting potential therapeutic modulation of SSC niche properties [125]. Empirical investigations have revealed noteworthy indications of compromised Leydig cell performance in males with a record of unexplained male infertility. This could be attributed to potential disturbances in the paracrine communication between the seminiferous epithelium and Leydig cells, or congenital dysfunction affecting both of these essential components [126]. Furthermore, within a mouse model, it was observed that the generation of glial cell line-derived neurotrophic factor GDNF by peritubular myoid cells plays a crucial role in spermatogonial growth. This underscores the significance of the interaction among key components of the spermatogonial stem cell niche, including Leydig cells and peritubular myoid cells, given that testosterone stimulates the expression of GDNF [118].

11. Challenges and future directions

11.1 The importance of optimizing cell isolation, transplantation techniques, and immunosuppression protocols

NOA, a condition characterized by low or absent sperm production, poses a significant challenge in male infertility. However, advancements in gene editing and combination therapies hold promise for its future treatment. Possible directions include:

1. *Gene editing to correct genetic defects*: CRISPR-Cas9, a gene editing tool, could correct specific genetic defects linked to NOA, potentially restoring normal sperm production [127].

2. *Induced pluripotent stem cell therapy*: iPSCs, reprogrammed adult cells, can transform into different cell types, including sperm cells. Scientists are investigating iPSCs for generating functional sperm in the lab, potentially offering a sperm source for individuals with NOA [128].

3. *Testicular sperm extraction (TESE) combined with assisted reproductive techniques*: TESE, which surgically retrieves sperm from the testicles, can be coupled with assisted reproductive methods like ICSI to facilitate egg fertilization and embryo transfer. This approach exhibits potential for successful pregnancies in certain instances of NOA [129].

4. Hormonal therapies: Hormonal treatments, including FSH and hCG, can boost sperm production in those with NOA, though their effectiveness varies by case [130].

5. *Combination therapies*: Combining various treatments can improve outcomes for NOA by addressing underlying causes and boosting sperm production. This may involve gene editing, hormonal therapies, and assisted reproductive techniques [131].

11.2 Ethical considerations and regulatory framework

Cell-based therapies, incorporating embryonic stem cells and genetic alterations, prompt significant ethical scrutiny. Key ethical aspects include:

1. *Respect for human life*: A central ethical concern pertains to the moral status of embryos, particularly in the context of embryonic stem cell research. Extracting these cells often entails destroying human embryos, prompting debates on whether this constitutes the loss of potential human life. This raises ethical questions about the treatment and utilization of human embryos in scientific or therapeutic endeavors [132].

2. *Informed consent*: Ethical concerns in cell-based therapies encompass securing informed consent, especially for embryonic stem cell use and genetic modifications. These techniques bear significant implications for individuals and their offspring. Clear communication of potential risks and benefits empowers informed decision-making by participants [133].

3. *Equity and access*: The ethical concerns surrounding cell-based therapies encompass equity and accessibility. These treatments are intricate and expensive, posing barriers for some. Ensuring fair access is vital to prevent worsening health disparities and promote healthcare justice.

4. *Genetic modifications and enhancement*: Genetic modifications raise ethical questions regarding the differentiation between therapeutic interventions and enhancements. They can address genetic disorders or enhance traits, leading to ongoing ethical debates and the need to define ethical boundaries [134].

5. *Long-term consequences and unintended effects*: Long-term implications and unintended outcomes of cell-based therapies, including genetic modifications, require thorough evaluation. Ethical responsibility necessitates rigorous research, safety assessments, and continuous monitoring to mitigate potential harm and unforeseen consequences for future generations.

6. *Regulatory oversight*: To address the complexity and risks of cell-based therapies, establishing effective regulatory frameworks is vital. Ethical concerns require the creation of strong regulations and oversight systems to ensure the ethical and responsible application of these technologies. Regulatory authorities must aim for a balance between innovation, patient safety, and public confidence to prevent unethical conduct and safeguard individuals' well-being [135].

11.3 The existing regulatory framework and guidelines for the clinical application of cell-based therapies in reproductive medicine

As of September 2021, I can discuss the regulatory framework and guidelines for using cell-based therapies in reproductive medicine. Keep in mind that these rules may change, so consult current sources and regulatory bodies for updates.

Many countries have government agencies that oversee cell-based therapies in reproductive medicine to ensure safety, efficacy, and ethical use. Here are key points about these regulations and guidelines:

1. *Regulatory authorities*: Various countries have specific regulatory agencies overseeing cell-based therapies. In the United States, the FDA regulates these therapies, and in the European Union, the EMA is responsible for oversight [136].

2. *Classification of cell therapies*: Regulatory bodies classify cell-based therapies based on intended use, risk, and manufacturing methods. This classification dictates oversight and regulatory routes. Categories, like advanced therapy medicinal products (ATMPs) or biological products, vary by country but remain consistent in the general framework [137].

3. *Preclinical testing*: Cell-based therapies undergo preclinical evaluation to assess safety and efficacy before clinical trials. This involves lab research and animal testing to gather evidence on benefits and risks.

4. *Clinical trials*: Clinical trials assess cell-based therapy safety and efficacy in humans. Regulatory bodies mandate researchers to secure approval and adhere to precise trial guidelines, encompassing participant selection, informed consent, treatment administration, and data gathering [138].

5. *Good manufacturing practices (GMP)*: Cell-based therapies used in reproductive medicine are often subject to stringent manufacturing requirements to ensure their quality, consistency, and safety. GMP guidelines regulate various aspects of manufacturing, including facilities, personnel, equipment, documentation, and quality control.

6. *Ethical considerations*: Cell-based therapies in reproductive medicine may raise ethical concerns related to the source of cells, their manipulation, and the implications of their use. Regulatory frameworks often include guidelines or principles to address these ethical considerations, such as informed consent, privacy protection, and appropriate handling of human tissues [139].

12. Future perspectives

Infertility, a multifaceted condition encompassing genetic, environmental, physical, and psychological factors alongside issues in germ cell production and transmission, persists as a challenge. Assisted reproductive technology ART, notably IVF, has facilitated numerous births but raises concerns about patient and offspring well-being. This review delves into refractory infertility, its traits, and treatment approaches, with an emphasis on stem cell potential in treatment.

Stem cell therapies, due to their pluripotent capabilities, emerge as ART alternatives. Research explores their utility in enhancing infertility treatment. The review covers translational studies investigating stem cell-based treatments' mechanisms: direct differentiation and cytokine secretion, customized for specific conditions. For age-related or irreversible fertility problems, germ-line stem cells have induced active gamete production, and mesenchymal stem cells contribute to immunoregulation and organ restoration.

Notably, stem cell therapies are presently in preclinical stages, prompting ethical concerns and diverse opinions. To transition into clinical practice, meticulous, long-term planning, thorough assessments, and vigilant oversight are essential to ensure precision, excellence, and safety. Autologous stem cells, sourced from the patient, show promise for future clinical use due to their safety and immunogenicity benefits.

13. Conclusion

Cell-based therapy shows promise in addressing NOA, a condition marked by the absence of sperm in ejaculation due to testicular dysfunction. Traditional treatments have limitations, prompting exploration of cell-based approaches using SSCs or iPSCs to restore spermatogenesis. Animal studies demonstrate successful fertility restoration *via* SSC transplantation, while human research advances in isolating and characterizing human SSCs. Challenges persist in scaling human SSCs and optimizing iPSC differentiation. Further research is needed to overcome technical hurdles and ensure safety and sustained functionality of transplanted cells, potentially providing a novel NOA treatment option and fertility restoration.

Author details

Ahmed Atwa[1*], Serag Eldin I. Elbehairi[2,3], Sayed Bakry[1], Ahmed B.M. Mehany[1], Mahmoud Ashry[4], Hussam Askar[4] and Mohammad Y. Alfaifi[2]

1 Faculty of Science (Boys), Zoology Department, Al-Azhar University, Cairo, Egypt

2 Faculty of Science, Biology Department, King Khalid University, Abha, Saudi Arabia

3 Cell Culture Lab, Egyptian Organization for Biological Products and Vaccines (VACSERA Holding Company), Agouza, Giza, Egypt

4 Faculty of Science, Zoology Department, Al-Azhar University, Assuit, Egypt

*Address all correspondence to: ahmed.atwa@azhar.edu.eg

References

[1] Matzuk MM, Lamb DJ. The biology of infertility: Research advances and clinical challenges. Nature Medicine. 2008;**14**(11):1197-1213

[2] Uhlén M et al. Tissue-based map of the human proteome. Science. 2015;**347**(6220):1260419

[3] Zhang X et al. Embryo development and live birth resulted from artificial oocyte activation after microdissection testicular sperm extraction with ICSI in patients with non-obstructive azoospermia. Frontiers in Endocrinology. 2023;**14**:1123541

[4] Logan S, Anazodo A. The psychological importance of fertility preservation counseling and support for cancer patients. Acta Obstetricia et Gynecologica Scandinavica. 2019;**98**(5):583-597

[5] Kherraf Z-E et al. Whole-exome sequencing improves the diagnosis and care of men with non-obstructive azoospermia. The American Journal of Human Genetics. 2022;**109**(3):508-517

[6] Tournaye H, Krausz C, Oates RD. Novel concepts in the aetiology of male reproductive impairment. The Lancet Diabetes & Endocrinology. 2017;**5**(7):544-553

[7] Zhankina R et al. Mesenchymal stromal/stem cells and their exosomes for restoration of spermatogenesis in non-obstructive azoospermia: A systemic review. Stem Cell Research & Therapy. 2021;**12**(1):229

[8] Wosnitzer M, Goldstein M, Hardy MP. Review of Azoospermia. Spermatogenesis. 2014;**4**(1):e28218

[9] Oud MS et al. Validation and application of a novel integrated genetic screening method to a cohort of 1,112 men with idiopathic azoospermia or severe oligozoospermia. Human Mutation. 2017;**38**(11):1592-1605

[10] Gordetsky J, van Wijngaarden E, O'Brien J. Redefining abnormal follicle-stimulating hormone in the male infertility population. BJU International. 2012;**110**(4):568-572

[11] Fernandez CJ, Chacko EC, Pappachan JM. Male obesity-related secondary hypogonadism—Pathophysiology, clinical implications and management. European Endocrinology. 2019;**15**(2):83-90

[12] Hammond GL. Sex hormone-binding globulin and the metabolic syndrome. In: Male Hypogonadism: Basic, Clinical and Therapeutic Principles. Cham: Springer International Publishing, Humana Press; 2017. pp. 305-324

[13] Hwang K et al. Evaluation of the azoospermic male: A committee opinion. Fertility and Sterility. 2018;**109**(5):777-782

[14] Peña VN, Kohn TP, Herati AS. Genetic mutations contributing to non-obstructive azoospermia. Best Practice & Research Clinical Endocrinology & Metabolism. 2020;**34**(6):101479

[15] Sharlip ID et al. Best practice policies for male infertility. Fertility and Sterility. 2002;**77**(5):873-882

[16] Corona G et al. Sperm recovery and ICSI outcomes in men with non-obstructive azoospermia: A systematic review and meta-analysis.

Human Reproduction Update. 2019;**25**(6):733-757

[17] Bucay N et al. A novel approach for the derivation of putative primordial germ cells and sertoli cells from human embryonic stem cells. Stem Cells. 2009;**27**(1):68-77

[18] Yang W et al. iPSC reprogramming from human peripheral blood using Sendai virus mediated gene transfer. International Journal of Biomedical and Health Sciences. 2021;**10**(4)

[19] Nayernia K et al. In vitro-differentiated embryonic stem cells give rise to male gametes that can generate offspring mice. Developmental Cell. 2006;**11**(1):125-132

[20] El-Sayed ME et al. Mesenchymal stem cell transplantation in burn wound healing: Uncovering the mechanisms of local regeneration and tissue repair. Histochemistry and Cell Biology. 2023

[21] Roshandel E et al. Cell-based therapy approaches in treatment of non-obstructive azoospermia. Reproductive Sciences. 2023;**30**(5):1482-1494

[22] Kim HJ, Park JS. Usage of human mesenchymal stem cells in cell-based therapy: Advantages and disadvantages. Development & Reproduction. 2017;**21**(1):1-10

[23] Jarrige M et al. The future of regenerative medicine: Cell therapy using pluripotent stem cells and acellular therapies based on extracellular vesicles. Cells. 2021;**10**. DOI: 10.3390/cells10020240

[24] Atwa A et al. Biodegradable materials from natural origin for tissue engineering and stem cells technologies. In: Ali GAM, Makhlouf ASH, editors. Handbook of Biodegradable Materials. Cham: Springer International Publishing; 2022. pp. 1-40

[25] Sampogna G, Guraya SY, Forgione A. Regenerative medicine: Historical roots and potential strategies in modern medicine. Journal of Microscopy and Ultrastructure. 2015;**3**(3):101-107

[26] Ashry M et al. Hormonal and inflammatory modulatory effects of hesperidin in hyperthyroidism-modeled rats. Frontiers in Immunology. 2023;**14**:1087397. DOI: 10.3389/fimmu.2023.1087397

[27] Ratcliffe E, Thomas RJ, Williams D. Current understanding and challenges in bioprocessing of stem cell-based therapies for regenerative medicine. British Medical Bulletin. 2011;**100**(1):137

[28] Robinson M et al. Human in vitro spermatogenesis as a regenerative therapy — Where do we stand? Nature Reviews Urology. 2023

[29] Chowdhury S et al. Stem cells an overview. Stem Cells: Biology and Therapeutics. 2021:1-21

[30] Kawasaki H et al. Current status and legal/ethical problems in the research use of the tissues of aborted human fetuses in Japan. Congenital Anomalies. 2020;**60**(6):166-174

[31] Ozawa H, Matsumoto T, Nakagawa M. Culturing human pluripotent stem cells for regenerative medicine. Expert Opinion on Biological Therapy. 2023:1-11

[32] Cullen I, Muneer A. Surgical sperm retrieval and MicroTESE. In: Allahbadia GN et al., editors. Textbook of Assisted Reproduction. Singapore: Springer Singapore; 2020. pp. 193-202

[33] Kang C, Punjani N, Schlegel PN. Reproductive chances of men with azoospermia due to spermatogenic dysfunction. Journal of Clinical Medicine. 2021;**10**:1400. DOI: 10.3390/jcm10071400

[34] Deng C-C, Liu G-H. Stem cell therapy for non-obstructive azoospermia. Zhonghua nan ke xue = National Journal of Andrology. 2020;**26**(4):351-356

[35] Tamadon A et al. Mesenchymal stem cell therapy of male infertility. In: Male Reproductive Health. 2019. p. 105

[36] Yan G et al. Ectopic expression of DAZL gene in goat bone marrow-derived mesenchymal stem cells enhances the trans-differentiation to putative germ cells compared to the exogenous treatment of retinoic acid or bone morphogenetic protein 4 signalling molecules. Cell Biology International. 2015;**39**(1):74-83

[37] Salem M et al. Germ cell differentiation of bone marrow mesenchymal stem cells. Andrologia. 2019;**51**(4):e13229

[38] Hajihoseini M et al. Induction of spermatogenesis after stem cell therapy of azoospermic Guinea pigs. Veterinary Archives. 2017;**87**(3):333-350

[39] Tamadon A et al. Induction of spermatogenesis by bone marrow-derived mesenchymal stem cells in busulfan-induced azoospermia in hamster. International Journal of Stem Cells. 2015;**8**(2):134-145

[40] Kadam P et al. Co-transplantation of mesenchymal stem cells improves spermatogonial stem cell transplantation efficiency in mice. Stem Cell Research & Therapy. 2018;**9**(1):317

[41] Atwa A, Mansour AM, Bakry S. Mesenchymal stem cells restore fertility in induced azoospermic rats following chemotherapy administration. Journal of Reproduction and Infertility. 2014;**5**(2):52-60

[42] Schuppe HC et al. Chronic orchitis: A neglected cause of male infertility? Andrologia. 2008;**40**(2):84-91

[43] Sanou I et al. Spermatogonial stem cell-based therapies: Taking preclinical research to the next level. Frontiers in Endocrinology. 2022;**13**

[44] Kanatsu-Shinohara M et al. Functional assessment of self-renewal activity of male germline stem cells following cytotoxic damage and serial transplantation1. Biology of Reproduction. 2003;**68**(5):1801-1807

[45] Valli H, Gassei K, Orwig KE. Stem cell therapies for male infertility: Where are we now and where are we going? Biennial Review of Infertility. 2015;**4**:17-39

[46] Forbes CM, Flannigan R, Schlegel PN. Spermatogonial stem cell transplantation and male infertility: Current status and future directions. Arab Journal of Urology. 2018;**16**(1):171-180

[47] Pourmoghadam Z et al. Current approaches for the treatment of male infertility with stem cell therapy. Journal of Cellular Physiology. 2018;**233**(10):6455-6469

[48] Seandel M et al. Generation of functional multipotent adult stem cells from GPR125+ germline progenitors. Nature Medicine. 2007;**449**(7160):346-350

[49] Phillips BT, Gassei K, Orwig KE. Spermatogonial stem cell regulation

and spermatogenesis. Philosophical Transactions of the Royal Society B: Biological Sciences. 2010;**365**(1546):1663-1678

[50] Park JE et al. Development of a three-dimensional hydrogel system for the maintenance of porcine spermatogonial stem cell self-renewal. Jet. 2017;**32**(4):343-351

[51] Freeman B. The active migration of germ cells in the embryos of mice and men is a myth. Reproduction-Cambridge. 2003;**125**(5):635-643

[52] Møllgård K et al. Human primordial germ cells migrate along nerve fibers and Schwann cells from the dorsal hind gut mesentery to the gonadal ridge. Molecular Human Reproduction. 2010;**16**(9):621-631

[53] Cremades N et al. In-vitro maturation of round spermatids using co-culture on Vero cells. Human Reproduction. 1999;**14**(5):1287-1293

[54] Gul M et al. Review of injection techniques for spermatogonial stem cell transplantation. Human Reproduction Update. 2020;**26**(3):368-391

[55] Brinster RL, Zimmermann JW. Spermatogenesis following male germ-cell transplantation. Proceedings of the National Academy of Sciences. 1994;**91**(24):11298-11302

[56] Takashima S, Shinohara T. Culture and transplantation of spermatogonial stem cells. Stem Cell Research. 2018;**29**:46-55

[57] Hermann BP et al. Spermatogonial stem cell transplantation into rhesus testes regenerates spermatogenesis producing functional sperm. Cell Stem Cell. 2012;**11**(5):715-726

[58] Shetty G et al. Postpubertal spermatogonial stem cell transplantation restores functional sperm production in rhesus monkeys irradiated before and after puberty. Andrology. 2021;**9**(5):1603-1616

[59] Radford JA. Is prevention of sterility possible in men? Annals of Oncology. 2000;**11**(Suppl 3):173-174

[60] Nagano MC. Homing efficiency and proliferation kinetics of male germ line stem cells following transplantation in mice. Biology of Reproduction. 2003;**69**(2):701-707

[61] Mirzapour T et al. Xenotransplantation assessment: Morphometric study of human spermatogonial stem cells in recipient mouse testes. Andrologia. 2015;**47**(6):626-633

[62] Dobrinski I et al. Computer assisted image analysis to assess colonization of recipient seminiferous tubules by spermatogonial stem cells from transgenic donor mice. Molecular Reproduction and Development. 1999;**53**(2):142-148

[63] Kanatsu-Shinohara M et al. Long-term proliferation in culture and germline transmission of mouse male germline stem cells. Biology of Reproduction. 2003;**69**(2):612-616

[64] Sadri-Ardekani H et al. Propagation of human spermatogonial stem cells In vitro. JAMA. 2009;**302**(19):2127-2134

[65] Sadri-Ardekani H et al. In vitro propagation of human prepubertal spermatogonial stem cells. JAMA. 2011;**305**(23):2416-2418

[66] Kossack N et al. A combined approach facilitates the reliable detection of human spermatogonia

in vitro. Human Reproduction. 2013;**28**(11):3012-3025

[67] Struijk RB et al. ITGA6+ human testicular cell populations acquire a mesenchymal rather than germ cell transcriptional signature during long-term culture. International Journal of Molecular Sciences. 2020:21. DOI: 10.3390/ijms21218269

[68] Baert Y et al. Orthotopic grafting of cryopreserved prepubertal testicular tissue: In search of a simple yet effective cryopreservation protocol. Fertility and Sterility. 2012;**97**(5):1152-1157

[69] McCoy DE et al. Structural absorption by barbule microstructures of super black bird of paradise feathers. Nature Communications. 2018;**9**(1):1

[70] Guo F et al. The transcriptome and DNA methylome landscapes of human primordial germ cells. Cell. 2015;**161**(6):1437-1452

[71] Sara Di P et al. EGR4-dependent decrease of UTF1 is associated with failure to reserve spermatogonial stem cells in infertile men. bioRxiv. 2021:2021.02.02.429371

[72] Di Persio S et al. Spermatogonial kinetics in humans. Development. 2017;**144**(19):3430-3439

[73] Sohni A et al. The neonatal and adult human testis defined at the single-cell level. Cell Reports. 2019;**26**(6):1501-1517.e4

[74] Jetten AM, Kang HS, Takeda Y. Retinoic acid-related orphan receptors α and γ: Key regulators of lipid/glucose metabolism, inflammation, and insulin sensitivity. Frontiers in Endocrinology. 2013;**4**:1

[75] Voigt AL et al. Metabolic requirements for spermatogonial stem cell establishment and maintenance In vivo and In vitro. International Journal of Molecular Sciences. 2021;**22**. DOI: 10.3390/ijms22041998

[76] Murdock MH et al. Human testis extracellular matrix enhances human spermatogonial stem cell survival In vitro. Tissue Engineering Part A. 2018;**25**(7-8):663-676

[77] Kurek M et al. Spermatogonia loss correlates with LAMA 1 expression in human prepubertal testes stored for fertility preservation. Cells. 2021;**10**(2)

[78] de Michele F et al. Preserved seminiferous tubule integrity with spermatogonial survival and induction of Sertoli and Leydig cell maturation after long-term organotypic culture of prepubertal human testicular tissue. Human Reproduction. 2017;**32**(1):32-45

[79] Nayernia K et al. Derivation of male germ cells from bone marrow stem cells. Laboratory Investigation. 2006;**86**(7):654-663

[80] Aboul Fotouh GI et al. Histological study on the protective effect of endogenous stem cell mobilization in busulfan-induced testicular injury in albino rats. Journal of Microscopy and Ultrastructure. 2018;**6**(4):197-204

[81] Alfano M et al. Anti-Mullerian hormone-to-testosterone ratio is predictive of positive sperm retrieval in men with idiopathic non-obstructive azoospermia. Scientific Reports. 2017;**7**(1):17638

[82] Menkveld R. Clinical significance of the low normal sperm morphology value as proposed in the fifth edition of the WHO Laboratory manual for the examination and processing of human semen. Asian Journal of Andrology. 2010;**12**(1):47-58

[83] Gandini L et al. Effect of chemo- or radiotherapy on sperm parameters of testicular cancer patients. Human Reproduction. 2006;**21**(11):2882-2889

[84] Chen X, Liang M, Wang D. Progress on the study of the mechanism of busulfan cytotoxicity. Cytotechnology. 2018;**70**:497-502

[85] Durairajanayagam D, Agarwal A, Ong C. Causes, effects and molecular mechanisms of testicular heat stress. Reproductive Biomedicine Online. 2015;**30**(1):14-27

[86] Azizollahi S et al. Recruiting testicular torsion introduces an azoospermic mouse model for spermatogonial stem cell transplantation. Urology Journal. 2014;**11**(3):1648-1655

[87] Abuelhija M et al. Rat models of post-irradiation recovery of spermatogenesis: Interstrain differences. Andrology. 2013;**1**(2):206-215

[88] Absalan F, Movahedin M, Mowla SJ. Evaluation of apoptotic genes expression and its protein after treatment of cryptorchid mice. Iranian Biomedical Journal. 2012;**16**(2):77-83

[89] Mobarak H et al. Intratesticular versus intraperitoneal injection of busulfan for the induction of azoospermia in a rat model. BMC Pharmacology and Toxicology. 2022;**23**(1):50

[90] Andersson BS et al. Clofarabine ± fludarabine with once daily i.v. busulfan as pretransplant conditioning therapy for advanced myeloid leukemia and MDS. Biology of Blood and Marrow Transplantation. 2011;**17**(6):893-900

[91] Gooptu M et al. A comparison of the myeloablative conditioning regimen fludarabine/busulfan with cyclophosphamide/total body irradiation, for allogeneic stem cell transplantation in the modern era: A cohort analysis. Biology of Blood and Marrow Transplantation. 2018;**24**(8):1733-1740

[92] Gayoso J et al. Busulfan-based myeloablative conditioning regimens for haploidentical transplantation in high-risk acute leukemias and myelodysplastic syndromes. European Journal of Haematology. 2018;**101**(3):332-339

[93] Chi H et al. Effect of genistein administration on the recovery of spermatogenesis in the busulfan-treated rat testis. Clinical and Experimental Reproductive Medicine. 2013;**40**(2):60-66

[94] Suttorp M, Millot F. Treatment of pediatric chronic myeloid leukemia in the year 2010: Use of tyrosine kinase inhibitors and stem-cell transplantation. Hematology. 2010;**2010**(1):368-376

[95] Ghasemi FM et al. Effect of melatonin on proliferative activity and apoptosis in spermatogenic cells in mouse under chemotherapy. Journal of Reproduction and Contraception. 2010;**21**(2):79-94

[96] Ogawa T, Dobrinski I, Brinster R. Recipient preparation is critical for spermatogonial transplantation in the rat. Tissue and Cell Biology International. 1999;**31**(5):461-472

[97] Kanatsu-Shinohara M et al. Germline niche transplantation restores fertility in infertile mice. Human Reproduction. 2005;**20**(9):2376-2382

[98] Kurkure P et al. Very small embryonic-like stem cells (VSELs) detected in azoospermic testicular biopsies of adult survivors of childhood

cancer. Reproductive Biology and Endocrinology. 2015;**13**:122

[99] Hjollund NH et al. Diurnal scrotal skin temperature and semen quality. The Danish First Pregnancy Planner Study Team. International Journal of Andrology. 2000;**23**(5):309-318

[100] Wang C et al. Effect of increased scrotal temperature on sperm production in normal men. Fertility and Sterility. 1997;**68**(2):334-339

[101] Mieusset R, Bengoudifa B, Bujan L. Effect of posture and clothing on scrotal temperature in fertile men. Journal of Andrology. 2007;**28**(1):170-175

[102] Chowdhury AK, Steinberger E. Early changes in the germinal epithelium of rat testes following exposure to heat. Journal of Reproduction and Fertility. 1970;**22**(2):205-212

[103] Munkelwitz R, Gilbert BR. Are boxer shorts really better? A critical analysis of the role of underwear type in male subfertility. The Journal of Urology. 1998;**160**(4):1329-1333

[104] Jensen TK et al. Inhibin B as a serum marker of spermatogenesis: Correlation to differences in sperm concentration and follicle-stimulating hormone levels. A study of 349 Danish men. The Journal of Clinical Endocrinology and Metabolism. 1997;**82**(12):4059-4063

[105] Hjollund NH et al. The relation between daily activities and scrotal temperature. Reproductive Toxicology. 2002;**16**(3):209-214

[106] Shiraishi K, Matsuyama H, Takihara H. Pathophysiology of varicocele in male infertility in the era of assisted reproductive technology. International Journal of Urology. 2012;**19**(6):538-550

[107] Carlsen E et al. History of febrile illness and variation in semen quality. Human Reproduction. 2003;**18**(10):2089-2092

[108] Lue YH et al. Single exposure to heat induces stage-specific germ cell apoptosis in rats: Role of intratesticular testosterone on stage specificity. Endocrinology. 1999;**140**(4):1709-1717

[109] Zhang M et al. Autophagy and apoptosis act as partners to induce germ cell death after heat stress in mice. PLoS One. 2012;**7**(7):e41412

[110] Fijak M et al. Infectious, inflammatory and 'autoimmune' male factor infertility: How do rodent models inform clinical practice? Human Reproduction Update. 2018;**24**(4):416-441

[111] Hasan H et al. Mechanism of inflammatory associated impairment of sperm function, spermatogenesis and steroidogenesis. Frontiers in Endocrinology. 2022;**13**:897029

[112] Pröbstl C et al. Immune cell characterization in spontaneous autoimmune orchitis in dogs. Theriogenology. 2022;**187**:219-226

[113] Nieschlag E et al. Disorders at the testicular level. Andrology: Male Reproductive Health Dysfunction. 2010:193-238

[114] Nicolas N et al. Testicular activin and follistatin levels are elevated during the course of experimental autoimmune epididymo-orchitis in mice. Scientific Reports. 2017;7:42391

[115] Rusz A et al. Influence of urogenital infections and inflammation on semen quality and male fertility. World Journal of Urology. 2012;**30**(1):23-30

[116] Abdallah AE et al. Immunomodulatory quinazoline-based thalidomide analogs: Design, synthesis, apoptosis and anticancer evaluations. Journal of Molecular Structure. 2023;**1281**:135164

[117] Agarwal A et al. Male infertility. The Lancet Diabetes & Endocrinology. 2021;**397**(10271):319-333

[118] Sagaradze G et al. Regenerative medicine for male infertility: A focus on stem cell niche injury models. Biomedical Journal. 2022;**45**(4):607-614

[119] Gunes S et al. The role of epigenetics in idiopathic male infertility. Journal of Assisted Reproduction. 2016;**33**:553-569

[120] Luján S et al. Sperm DNA methylation epimutation biomarkers for male infertility and FSH therapeutic responsiveness. Scientific Reports. 2019;**9**(1):16786

[121] Salas-Huetos A et al. The role of miRNAs in male human reproduction: A systematic review. Andrology. 2020;**8**(1):7-26. Epub 2019/10/04. DOI: 10.1111/andr.12714

[122] Kothandaraman N et al. Pathogenic landscape of idiopathic male infertility: New insight towards its regulatory networks. NPJ Genomic Medicine. 2016;**1**(1):1-9

[123] Razavi SM et al. Comprehensive functional enrichment analysis of male infertility. Scientific Reports. 2017;**7**(1)

[124] Bansal SK et al. Differential genes expression between fertile and infertile spermatozoa revealed by transcriptome analysis. PLoS One. 2015;**10**(5):e0127007

[125] Zhao LY et al. Single-cell analysis of developing and azoospermia human testicles reveals central role of Sertoli cells. Nature. Communications. 2020;**11**(1)

[126] Andersson AM et al. Impaired Leydig cell function in infertile men: A study of 357 idiopathic infertile men and 318 proven fertile controls. Journal of Clinical Endocrinology and Metabolism. 2004;**89**(7):3161-3167

[127] Cinà DP, Phillips D, Flannigan R. CRISPR/Cas9 in male factor infertility. Current Tissue Microenvironment Reports. 2020;**1**(3):89-97

[128] Liu J et al. Generation and characterization of reprogrammed sheep induced pluripotent stem cells. Theriogenology. 2012;**77**(2):338-346 e1

[129] Aydos K, Aydos OS. Sperm selection procedures for optimizing the outcome of ICSI in patients with NOA. Journal of Clinical Medicine. 2021;**10**(12):2687

[130] Kim D et al. Long-acting recombinant human follicle-stimulating hormone (SAFA-FSH) enhances spermatogenesis. Frontiers in Endocrinology. 2023;**14**:1132172

[131] Assidi M. Infertility in men: Advances towards a comprehensive and integrative strategy for precision theranostics. Cell. 2022;**11**(10):1711

[132] Sivaraman MAF. Ethical guiding principles of "do no harm" and the "intention to save lives" in relation to human embryonic stem cell research: Finding common ground between religious views and principles of medical ethics. Asian Bioethics Review. 2019;**11**(4):409-435

[133] de Jongh D et al. Early-phase clinical trials of bio-artificial organ technology: A systematic review of ethical issues. Transplant International. 2022;**35**:10751

[134] Macpherson I, Roqué MV, Segarra I. Ethical challenges of germline genetic enhancement. Frontiers in Genetics. 2019;**10**:767

[135] Manghwar H et al. CRISPR/Cas systems in genome editing: Methodologies and tools for sgRNA design, off-target evaluation, and strategies to mitigate off-target effects. Advanced Science. 2020;**7**(6):1902312

[136] Von Tigerstrom B. Revising the regulation of stem cell-based therapies: Critical assessment of potential models. Food and Drug. 2015;**70**:315

[137] Laurencin CT, McClinton A. Regenerative cell-based therapies: Cutting edge, bleeding edge, and off the edge. Regenerative Engineering and Translational Medicine. 2020;**6**:78-89

[138] Rayment EA, Williams DJ. Concise review: Mind the gap: Challenges in characterizing and quantifying cell-and tissue-based therapies for clinical translation. Stem Cells. 2010;**28**(5):996-1004

[139] Najar M et al. Mesenchymal stromal cell-based therapy: New perspectives and challenges. Journal of Clinical Medicine. 2019;**8**(5):626

Chapter 5

Advances in Male Infertility Treatment through Assisted Reproductive Technology

Murid Javed and Seang L. Tan

Abstract

Male infertility is responsible for 40–50% of human infertility. Earlier treatment options for male factor infertility included timed intercourse, intrauterine insemination, or *in vitro* fertilization. These techniques are not helpful in severe male factor infertility cases as either the sperm number is extremely low or sperm motility is very poor. The introduction of intracytoplasmic sperm injection has opened the door for numerous advancements as only one sperm is needed for one egg. It has enabled men with few or no sperm in their ejaculates to have their own offspring. Surgical sperm retrieval techniques, with or without the help of a microscope, have been invented to retrieve sperm from the epididymis or testicular tissue. The clinical outcomes after the utilization of these techniques are similar to those obtained after the use of ejaculated sperm. Preimplantation genetic tests are now available to detect chromosomal aneuploidies, single gene defects, or chromosomal structural rearrangements in embryos created by using normal or defective sperm or eggs. This chapter explains in a comprehensible way, the basic and the more advanced assisted reproductive technologies to treat male factor infertility.

Keywords: male infertility, sperm, IVF, ICSI, PESA, TESA, TESE, micro-TESE, PGT

1. Introduction

Infertility is an inability to achieve pregnancy after one year of unprotected sex. It can be due to male factors, female factors or their combination. Male factor infertility can be treated with medicines or utilization of assisted reproductive technologies. The effects of medicines or hormones on sperm production or quality are noticeable after about 90 days as it takes this much time to observe new sperm population. The assisted reproductive technologies, on the other hand, make use of existing levels of sperm production and provide immediate solutions that could be simple washing or concentrating sperm for intra-uterine insemination (IUI), in vitro fertilization (IVF) or intracytoplasmic sperm injection (ICSI). After the advent of ICSI, only one sperm is needed to fertilize an egg as compared to millions of sperm required for natural conception, IUI or IVF. For ICSI, the sperm can be processed by simple wash [1], density gradient [2], swim up [3], or by using newly introduced devices like Microfluidic [4, 5] or Zymote [6]. Ejaculated, surgically collected, fresh or cryopreserved sperm have been used successfully. This chapter will explain basic and advanced assisted reproductive technologies to treat male factor infertility. The advanced scientific information is presented for easy understanding by a general reader. Those seeking in-depth knowledge are recommended to read the referenced articles.

2. Male reproductive organs

The male reproductive organs are shown in **Figure 1**. The sperm are produced in the testes and stored in the epididymis. At the time of ejaculation, the sperm are transported in a small quantity of fluid through the vas deference. The seminal

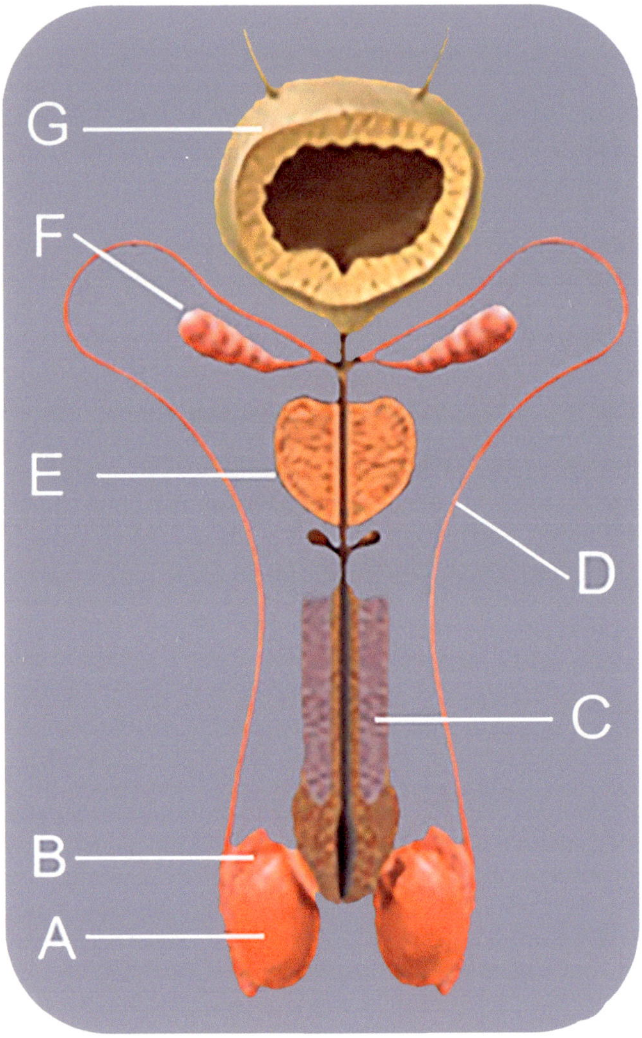

Figure 1.
Diagrammatic presentation of male reproductive organs. A = testis; B = epididymis; C = penis; D = vas deferens; E = prostate gland; F = bulbourethral gland; and G = urinary bladder. (the diagram is modified from Serono educational pamphlet).

vesicles and the prostate glands add their secretions to increase the seminal volume. The semen is then ejaculated through the urethra which is a common passage for the urine and the semen.

3. Advances in semen evaluation

Semen evaluation is required to determine male factor infertility. The laboratories have been performing semen analysis by manual microscopy [7, 8]. The determination of semen volume, sperm concentration, motility, and morphology are minimal requirements. These parameters can be accurately determined by manual microscopy; however, variations exist between different technologists and different labs. Computerized semen analysis [9, 10] was introduced to eliminate these variations and to determine additional sperm characteristics. The computer-assisted semen analysis systems have enabled partial automation of routine semen analysis. These systems can determine some semen parameters which cannot be determined by manual microscopy like the speed of sperm progression. They lacked wider acceptance [11] due to their complicated operation, high initial cost, expensive maintenance, and inability to analyze Micro-TESE and severe male factor samples. Newer and improved computer-assisted semen analyzers are gradually improving and entering the market to overcome these difficulties by integrating artificial intelligence optical microscopic technology [12].

The semen parameters are affected by days of abstinence, temperature at which semen is kept after ejaculation, and the time of evaluation after ejaculation. To avoid any deleterious effects and to get an accurate analysis, the production of semen at the treating facility is recommended. The lower reference limits for the most commonly assessed semen parameters are given in **Table 1**. These are usually considered standard semen values [13].

Determination of sperm DNA fragmentation is now becoming a routine. Abnormal expression of any functional gene in the process of spermatogenesis, maturation, and storage may affect sperm morphology, structure, or function, and induce male infertility. The sperm DNA integrity is crucial for fertilization, blastocyst formation, and the development of healthy offspring [14]. A number of tests are available for the detection of sperm DNA fragmentation [15]. Less than 30% sperm DNA fragmentation is generally acceptable and requires no medical intervention.

Sperm aneuploidy is associated with detrimental effects, particularly recurrent pregnancy loss. These sperm chromosomal abnormalities happen during meiosis or

Characteristic	Lower reference limit
Semen volume (ml)	1.5 (1.4–1.7)
Total sperm number (10^6 per ejaculate)	39 (33–46)
Sperm concentration (10^6 per ml)	15 (12–16)
Total motility (Progressive + non-progressive, %)	40 (38–42)
Progressive motility (%)	32 (31–34)
Sperm morphology (normal forms, %)	4 (3.0–4.0)

Table 1.
Lower reference limits (5th centiles and their 95% confidence intervals) for semen characteristics.

mitosis of sperm. Sperm aneuploidy is detected by fluorescent molecular probes for chromosomes 13, 18, 21, X, and Y [15]. This test is not widely available; therefore, fertility clinics rely on semen analysis, sperm DNA fragmentation test, and male karyotyping for the evaluation of male factor infertility.

Home-based semen analysis systems have also been introduced like Sperm Check Fertility and Micra Sperm Test [16, 17]. These tests only indicate whether further testing is needed or not, as many tests can only provide information on one or a few sperm parameters. Thus, these home base tests are not a replacement for semen analysis in a specialized laboratory.

4. Treatment options based on semen quality

The decision of a reproductive laboratory technique to treat male factor infertility is based on the results of basic semen evaluation, determination of sperm DNA fragmentation, sperm aneuploidy, semen culture and sensitivity, presence of round cells, and sperm agglutination. In the majority of men, semen evaluation on two different occasions, karyotyping and sperm DNA fragmentation test are enough. The most commonly adopted treatment pathway is given in **Figure 2**. The choice of treatment is determined by the specialist. The number of attempts and duration in between attempts is determined by the specialist and the couple. The success rates vary among treatment options and are described in the subsequent sections.

5. Timed intercourse

The specialist will monitor the menstrual cycle and determine the best time for the release of ova based on the ovarian follicular measurements and reproductive endocrine hormone profile to recommend the time for intercourse. The chance of achieving a clinical pregnancy after timed intercourse with ovulation prediction is about 9% [18]. The number of attempts of timed intercourse is dependent on the specialist and the couple. This procedure may be more helpful for couples with younger female ages and men with almost normal sperm parameters.

6. Intrauterine insemination (IUI)

Intrauterine insemination is a relatively cheaper, less intensive treatment as compared to IVF/ICSI, for achieving pregnancy [19]. Usually, the ovaries are stimulated with a low dose of follicle-stimulating hormone (FSH) to increase the number of follicles. The ovulation is triggered with human chorionic gonadotropin (hCG) for maturation and release of oocytes. On the day of IUI, semen produced from the male partner is washed, concentrated, and deposited in the uterine cavity for in vivo fertilization (**Figure 3**). Many variables may influence success rates after IUI. On average, pregnancy rates of 7.9–23% per IUI cycle have been reported [20]. Usually, more than three IUI attempts are not recommended as the cost of treatment exceeds than one attempt of IVF/ICSI, and the latter provides higher success rates.

Timed Intercourse (TIC)
The semen parameters are normal. There is no ejaculatory/intercourse problem

↓

Intra-uterine Insemination (IUI)
The sperm concentration is low; however, 5 million motile sperm are expected after the semen processing from one or combining 2 ejaculates. The progressive forward motility is good.

↓

In vitro Fertilization (IVF)
The sperm concentration is low and less than 1 million motile sperm are expected after processing the whole ejaculate. Three attempts of IUI have failed. The progressive forward motility is good.

↓

Intracytoplasmic Sperm Injection (ICSI)
One sperm is needed for one egg. Sperm from fresh/frozen-thawed sample, TESA, TESE, PESA , and micro-TESE can be used. Immotile, round headed, and abnormal morphology sperm can be used.

↓

ICSI with PGT
PGT can be combined with ICSI for selection of embryos with normal DNA. It is helpful in cases when abnormal karyotype/genetic defects are found, or in females >40 yrs.

Figure 2.
The most commonly adapted treatment pathway based on semen analysis. In this case, there is no apparent female factor infertility. The deficiency is found in semen characteristics.

7. In vitro fertilization (IVF)

In vitro fertilization is a process in which ovaries are stimulated to produce more follicles. Each ovarian follicle is expected to have one egg. The eggs are retrieved and fertilized *in vitro* (outside the body) by the addition of the appropriate number of sperm. **Figure 4** outlines the timeline for the IVF procedure. The period from point A to B takes several days depending on the protocol for ovarian stimulation. The eggs are usually collected 36 hours after administration of an injection that further grows and matures the eggs. The collected oocytes from ovarian follicles are given to the Embryology laboratory for their maintenance in appropriate culture conditions of temperature, humidity, gas, and nutrition. Usually, 3–4 eggs are placed in a petri dish and the appropriate number of processed sperm is added for IVF (**Figure 5**). The egg collection day is considered day-0. The fertilization is checked 16–19 hours after egg insemination and the culture is continued for up to 7 days. If the couple is undergoing fresh embryo transfer, one embryo at the blastocyst stage (day-5 to day-7) is transferred into the uterus for further growth inside the body. Extra embryos are cryopreserved for future use. The pregnancy test is performed 14 days after egg collection and the fetal heartbeat is checked from 42 to 56 days. If the embryo transfer is not successful, another attempt at frozen embryo transfer is performed after proper preparation of endometrium.

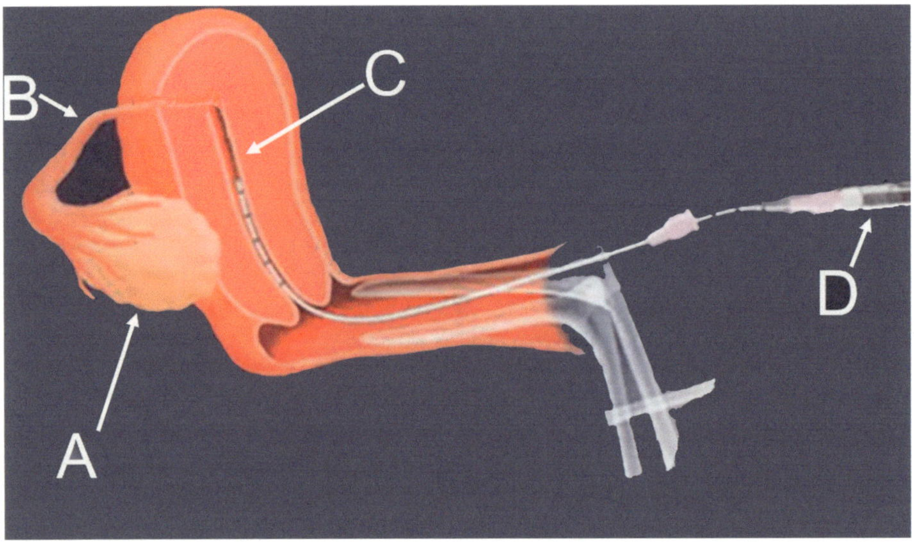

Figure 3.
Diagrammatic presentation of intrauterine insemination procedure. Semen from the male partner is washed, concentrated, and injected into the uterine cavity for in vivo fertilization. A = ovary; B = fallopian tube; C = uterine cavity; and D = a syringe attached to a catheter containing processed semen. (the diagram is modified from Serono educational pamphlet).

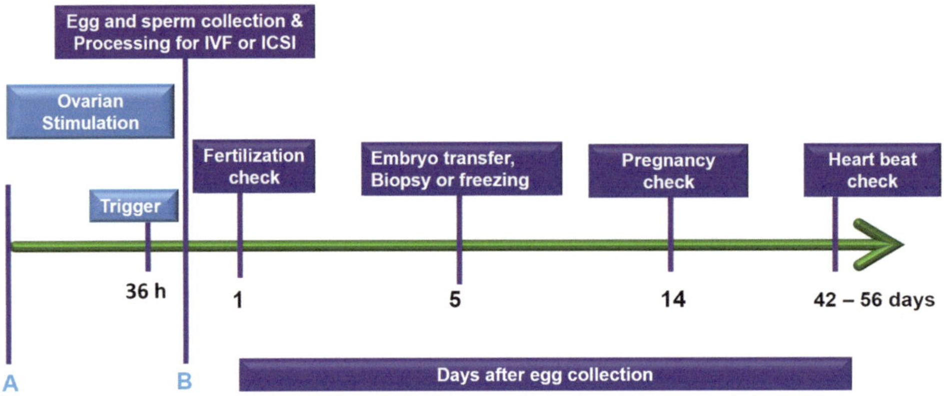

Figure 4.
Timeline for IVF or ICSI procedure starting from ovarian stimulation to the detection of fetal heartbeat.

With advancements in the technology, more options are available. These include; (1) performing embryo biopsy for genetic testing at the blastocyst stage (day-5 to day-7) and cryopreserving biopsied embryos, and (2) cryopreserving all embryos without biopsy for future use.

Depending on the quality of oocytes, sperm, or cause of infertility, about 50% of eggs fertilize. The chances of complete failed fertilization after IVF are 5–10% [21]. Couples who cannot take the risk of complete failed fertilization or want a higher number of eggs fertilized, prefer ICSI. The fertilization rate after ICSI among injected oocytes is significantly higher (72.3% ± 24.3%) than for IVF (59.2% ± 25.9%). However, complete failed fertilization still occurs after ICSI and the incidence is 1–3% [22, 23]. The good-quality embryo rate and clinical outcomes are not different

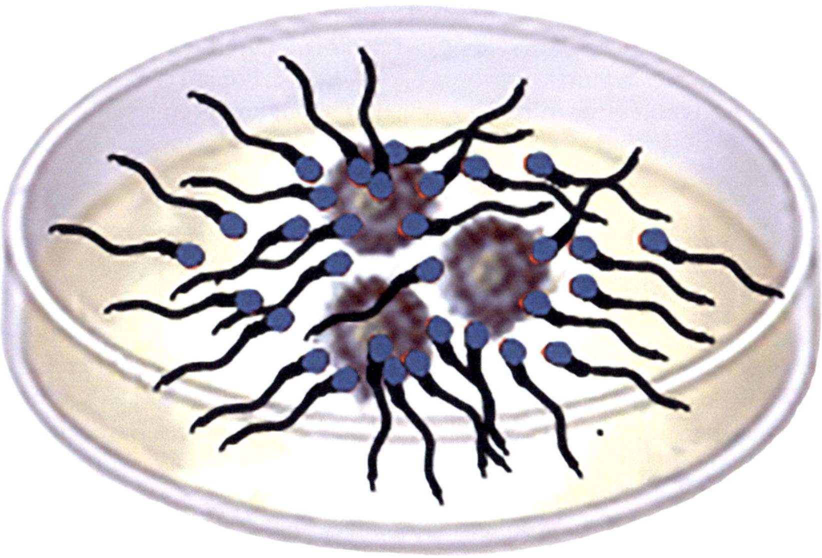

Figure 5.
In vitro fertilization in a petri dish. Usually, 3–4 eggs are placed in a petri dish and an appropriate number of sperm is added. The fertilization is checked 16–19 hours later.

between embryos from conventional IVF (16.6% ± 23.2%) and embryos from ICSI (16.6% ± 26.6%). Split fertilization (fertilizing some eggs with IVF and some with ICSI) decreases the risk of total fertilization failure. The assurance of fertilization with ICSI has gradually increased the use of ICSI [24] to the extent that many Embryology labs are performing 100% ICSI for all infertility cases.

The success after IVF varies significantly depending on the underlying infertility cause and the type of IVF treatment. The age of the female partner remains the most influential factor. During the initial years of IVF, most embryo transfers were performed on day-3 with multiple embryos, resulting in multiple pregnancies. The multiple pregnancies posed great risks to the mother and the developing fetuses. There has been a gradual transition from day-3 embryo transfer to day-5 embryo transfer with a single embryo to reduce the multiple births and to improve the pregnancy rate. Presently, almost all embryo transfers are performed at the blastocyst stage (day-5 to day-7) with a single embryo at each transfer.

The cumulative live-birth rate from up to six cycles of IVF in a study of more than 6000 patients undergoing 14,248 cycles was 51% with the conservative analysis and 72% with the optimistic analysis. The conservative analysis assumed that no live births happened among patients who did not return for subsequent IVF cycles and the optimistic analysis assumed that patients who did not return would have the same chance of a pregnancy resulting in a live birth as patients who continued treatment [25]. In another study, using freeze all strategy, the overall live birth rate of 50.74% in the first complete cycle among 20,687 women was achieved through IVF [26]. The complete cycle was defined as all the frozen-thawed embryo transfer attempts resulting from one round of ovarian stimulation. In this study, the live birth rate declined from 63.81% for women under 31 years of age to 4.71% for women over 40 years of age. The main cause of infertility in this study was tubal occlusion. The

IVF was performed in 66.38%, ICSI in 27.38%, and both IVF and ICSI in 6.24% of cycles. The IVF not only increases the success rate as compared to the IUI procedure but overcomes problems in female partners like blocked fallopian tubes. The IVF treatment often overcomes infertility in younger women; however, it does not reverse the age-dependent decline in fertility [25].

8. Intracytoplasmic sperm injection (ICSI)

In this technique, a sperm is injected directly into the cytoplasm of an egg. The processes of ovarian stimulation, egg collection, and culture are similar to the IVF procedure. The only difference is the fertilization process. For ICSI, after collection, the eggs are stripped of all cells surrounding the zona pellucida so that the egg maturity can be determined and sperm can be deposited accurately. Both sperm and eggs are microscopic structures, therefore very precisely made microscopic tools and a high-power inverted microscope are required (**Figure 6**).

For injection, the sperm is immobilized by an injection pipette (**Figure** 7 A) and aspirated into it (**Figure** 7 B). The egg is held in a desired position by a holding pipette and the injection pipette containing the sperm is inserted from the opposite end (**Figure** 7 C). The injection pipette is advanced further close to the opposite end of the egg (**Figure** 7 D). A small amount of cytoplasm is aspirated into the injection pipette to ensure egg membrane breakage. If the cytoplasm moves freely, the sperm is deposited there (**Figure** 7 E), and the injection needle is drawn out of the egg slowly (**Figure** 7 F).

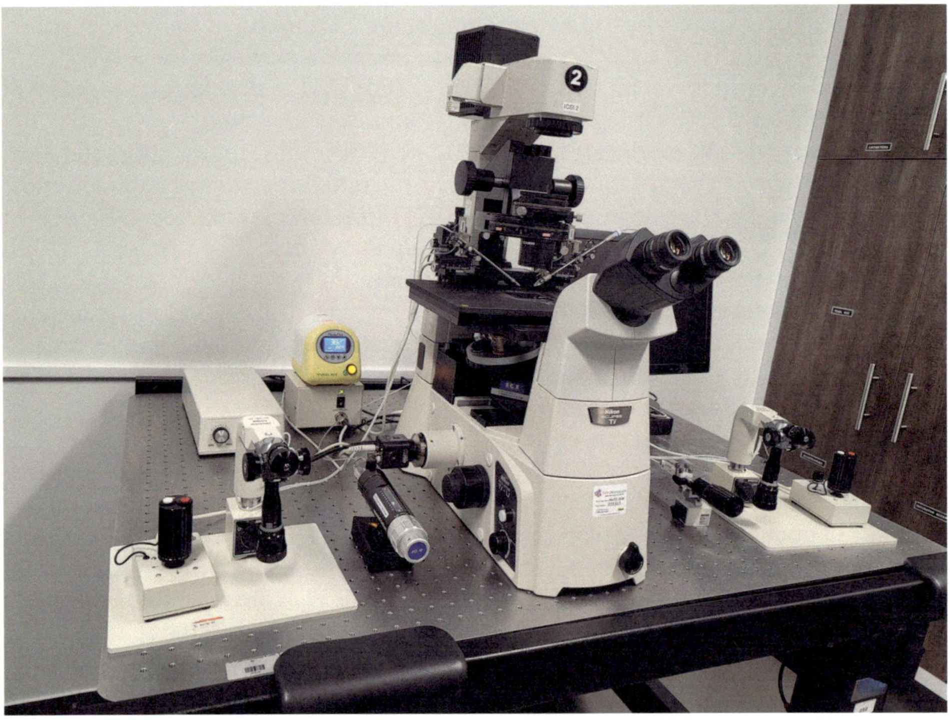

Figure 6.
Inverted microscope equipped with micro-tools for handling the egg and sperm and performing the ICSI procedure. A vibration free table is required to prevent damage to the egg during injection procedure.

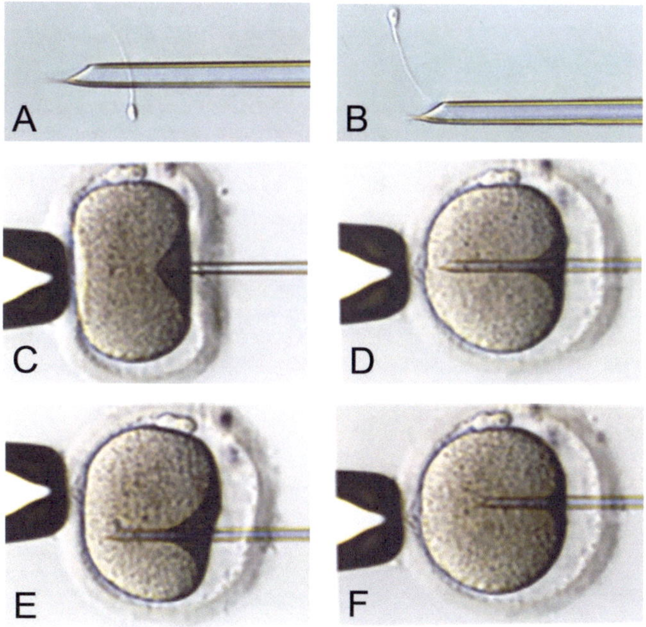

Figure 7.
ICSI steps. (A) the sperm is immobilized and its membrane broken by the injection pipette; (B) the sperm is aspirated into the injection pipette; (C) the egg is held by a holding pipette and the injection pipette is inserted through the zona pellucida into the egg cytoplasm from the opposite end; (D) the injection pipette is advanced further close to the opposite end of the egg; (E) a small amount of cytoplasm is aspirated into the injection pipette to ensure egg membrane breakage. If the cytoplasm moves freely, the sperm is deposited there; and (F) the injection needle is drawn out of egg slowly.

There are many situations, like severe male factor, globozoospermia, and azoospermia, for which fertilization by IVF cannot happen, therefore, the sperm has to be injected directly into the egg. For ICSI, only one sperm is needed for an egg, whereas, for IVF about 100, 000 motile sperm per 1 mL, and the IUI 5 million sperm per insemination are generally recommended. Because of this requirement of one sperm for one egg, many men with rare sperm in their ejaculate have been able to father their children. In men suffering from azoospermia (who have no sperm in their ejaculate), sperm can be retrieved from the epididymis or directly from the testis by different techniques.

Figure 8 explains different sites and techniques for obtaining sperm from male reproductive organs. The preferred, simple, and economical method for sperm availability is to have a male partner ejaculate a semen sample even in severe male factor infertility cases (**Figure 8**, H). The semen is diluted and mixed with appropriate media, centrifuged, supernatant removed, and only the 50 micro-liter pellet is examined to find enough sperm for the expected number of retrieved eggs. This procedure should be repeated multiple times before egg collection to obtain and freeze enough sperm for subsequent use on the day of egg collection.

If the sperm are not found from at least two ejaculates two weeks apart, the urologist's help is needed to obtain sperm from the epididymis. The procedure is called percutaneous epididymal sperm aspiration (PESA; **Figure 8**, J). If this procedure does not provide sperm, the testicular biopsy/testicular sperm aspiration (TESA; **Figure 8**, I) has to be performed by the urologist. The advanced options are testicular

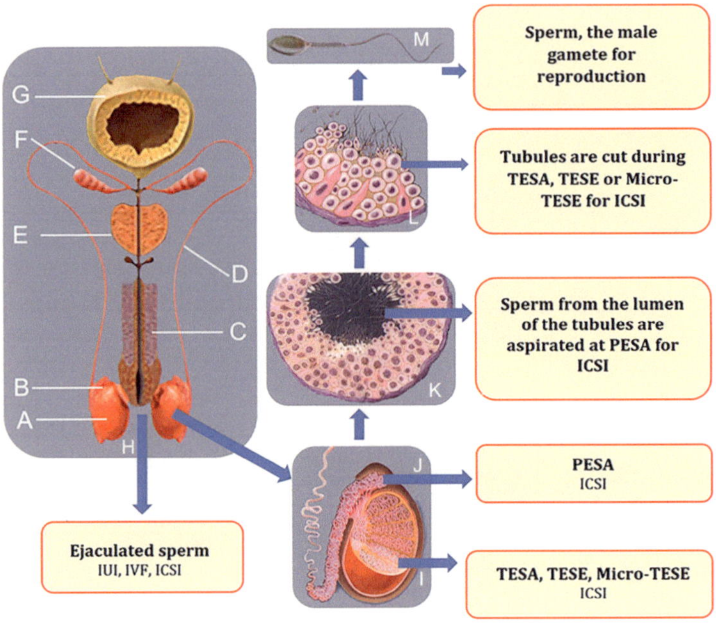

Figure 8.
Diagrammatic presentation of different sources of sperm for ICSI from male reproductive organs. The complexity of sperm retrieval depends on the site of collection and the type of retrieval procedure. The sperm are made in the seminiferous tubules of the testicles, stored in the epididymis, and transported by various ducts. Based on the source of sperm, appropriate assisted reproductive technique is applied. A = testicle, the site of spermatogenesis; B = epididymis, a place for sperm maturation and storage; C = penis, D = vas deference, a tube to transport sperm at ejaculation; E = prostate glands, adds their secretion to sperm; F = seminal vesicles, adds their secretion to sperm; G = urinary bladder; H = ejaculated sperm source; I = site for surgical sperm retrieval from testicular tissue; J = epididymis for sperm collection; K = microscopic structure of a tubule where the sperm are formed; L = a section of the tubule showing different cell types and progression from round cells to a flagellar cell (sperm); and M = a fully formed sperm. (the diagram is extracted from Serono educational pamphlet).

sperm extraction (TESE) without a microscope or Micro-TESE in which the testicular tissue is dissected under a microscope. In **Figure 8**, K and L are showing the testicular tubules where the sperm are formed.

Live births have been reported from fresh or frozen-thawed sperm retrieved by any of the above-mentioned techniques [27–29]. Pregnancy and delivery have been reported after the collection of only one egg, its ICSI, and the transfer of only one embryo [30].

Globozoospermia is a condition in which all or most of the sperm are round-headed. These sperm lack PLC zeta (PLCζ) which is required for oocyte activation and fertilization [31]. The round-headed sperm are unable to fertilize eggs. Fertilization of eggs with ICSI and artificial oocyte activation with calcium ionophore or other substances have solved this problem and many births have been reported [32, 33].

Another challenge in severe male factor infertility is the presence of all immotile sperm in the semen sample. Such sperm may be alive but not moving or could be dead. The sperm motility is due to its tail which is not required for fertilization by ICSI, however, injection of a viable sperm is desired. Also, frozen-thawed testicular sperm often lack motility. For such cases, techniques have been developed to differentiate between viable and non-viable sperm. Usually, the hypoosmotic swelling technique or addition of pentoxifylline/theophylline to the sperm preparation successfully differentiates between alive and dead sperm [34, 35].

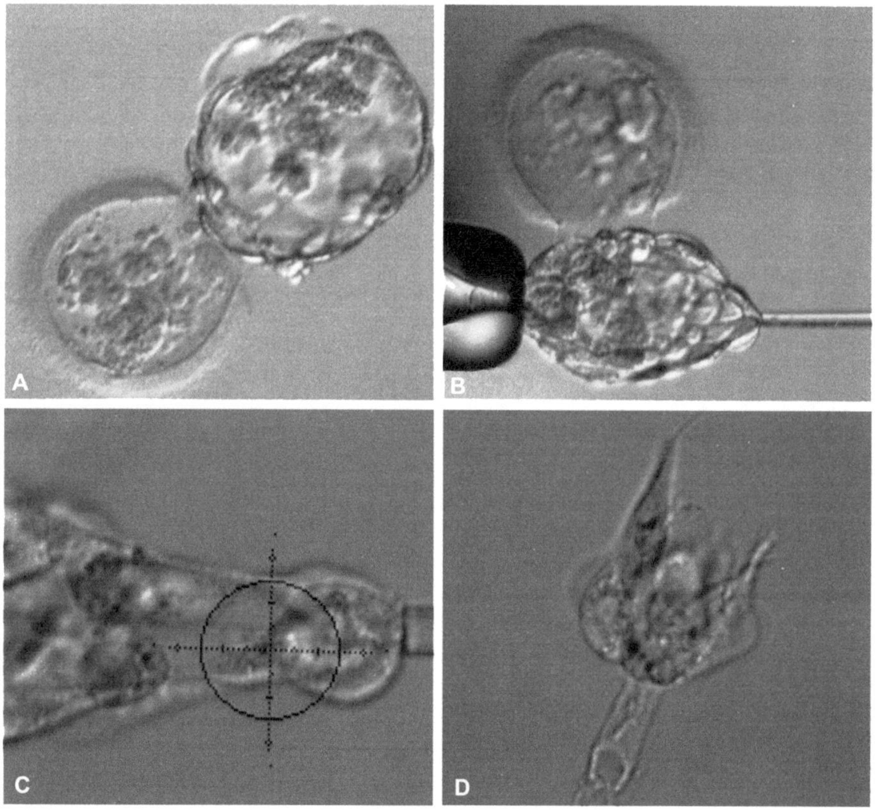

Figure 9.
Steps to perform embryo biopsy at the blastocyst stage. It is preferred that the biopsy is performed after the embryo has become a blastocyst but has not yet fully hatched. In this figure, the blastocyst is hatched (A). The trophectoderm is stretched out by a holding pipette on the left side and by a biopsy pipette on the right side (B and C). The stretched cells are cut by laser shots (C). A few (3–5) trophectodermal cells are sent to the genetic lab for genetic testing. The biopsied blastocyst is frozen.

9. IVF/ICSI with preimplantation genetic testing (PGT)

The difference between IVF/ICSI and IVF/ICSI with PGT is that at the blastocyst stage (day-5 to day-7), a few cells from the outer layer (trophectoderm) of each embryo are taken and sent to the genetic testing lab. The biopsied blastocysts are frozen and transferred a few months later based on genetic test results (**Figure 9**).

The blastocyst PGT is defined as a test that analyses the DNA from the trophectoderm of a blastocyst for HLA typing or for determining genetic abnormalities. There are 3 types of blastocyst PGT: PGT-A, is for the detection of chromosomal aneuploidies; PGT-M, is for the detection of monogenic/single gene defects and PGT-SR, is for the detection of chromosomal structural rearrangements [36].

Due to the new and safer embryo biopsy techniques and advancements in genetic testing, PGT-A has been widely practiced, with some clinics performing PGT-A for all infertile couples. The liberal use of this very expensive technology for all infertile couples is controversial [37, 38]. Several studies reported higher birth rates after PGT-A and elective single-euploid embryo transfer, though these studies have important limitations [39].

10. Conclusions

Assisted reproductive technologies have rapidly evolved over the past few decades and are providing significantly higher birth outcomes in all categories of infertile men. These techniques are safe and offer hope to many men wishing for a healthy child. The introduction of ICSI opened a new era and revolutionized the treatment of male factor infertility. The addition of surgical sperm retrieval techniques (PESA, TESA, TESE, and Micro-TESE) has further improved outcomes for male infertility. The newer genetic technologies (PGT-A, PGT-M, and PGT-SR provide assurance for the birth of a genetically normal child.

Acknowledgements

We acknowledge the graphic material provided by Serono Canada based on which some figures were designed.

Conflict of interest

The authors declare no conflict of interest.

Author details

Murid Javed* and Seang L. Tan
OriginElle Fertility Clinic and Women's Health Centre, Montreal, Canada

*Address all correspondence to: murid.javed@gmail.com

References

[1] Henkel RR, Schill WB. Sperm preparation for ART. Reproductive Biology and Endocrinology. 2003;**1**(1):1-22

[2] Quinn MM, Ribeiro S, Juarez-Hernandez F, Simbulan RK, Jalalian L, Cedars MI, et al. Microfluidic preparation of spermatozoa for ICSI produces similar embryo quality to density-gradient centrifugation: A pragmatic, randomized controlled trial. Human Reproduction. 2022;**37**(7):1406-1413

[3] Oguz Y, Guler I, Erdem A, Mutlu MF, Gumuslu S, Oktem M, et al. The effect of swim-up and gradient sperm preparation techniques on deoxyribonucleic acid (DNA) fragmentation in subfertile patients. Journal of Assisted Reproduction and Genetics. 2018;**35**:1083-1089

[4] Yetkinel S, Kilicdag EB, Aytac PC, Haydardedeoglu B, Simsek E, Cok T. Effects of the microfluidic chip technique in sperm selection for intracytoplasmic sperm injection for unexplained infertility: A prospective, randomized controlled trial. Journal of Assisted Reproduction and Genetics. 2019;**36**:403-409

[5] Vasilescu SA, Khorsandi S, Ding L, Bazaz SR, Nosrati R, Gook D, et al. A microfluidic approach to rapid sperm recovery from heterogeneous cell suspensions. Scientific Reports. 2021;**11**(1):1-1

[6] Anderson AR, Kasa E, Taylor D, Covington D, Williams E, Bhakta SA, et al. Euploidy rates and pregnancy outcomes using the Zymōt™ device for sperm preparation. Fertility and Sterility. 2020;**114**(3):e43-e44

[7] Andrade-Rocha FT. Semen analysis in laboratory practice: An overview of routine tests. Journal of Clinical Laboratory Analysis. 2003;**17**(6):247-258

[8] Douglas C, Parekh N, Kahn LG, Henkel R, Agarwal A. A novel approach to improving the reliability of manual semen analysis: A paradigm shift in the workup of infertile men. The World Journal of Men's Health. 2021;**39**(2):172

[9] Tomlinson MJ, Naeem A. CASA in the medical laboratory: CASA in diagnostic andrology and assisted conception. Reproduction, Fertility and Development. 2018;**30**(6):850-859

[10] Schardein JN, Fendereski K, Hotaling JM. Evolution of the basic semen analysis and processing sperm. Current Opinion in Urology. 2023;**33**(1):16-23

[11] Agarwal A, Henkel R, Huang CC, Lee MS. Automation of human semen analysis using a novel artificial intelligence optical microscopic technology. Andrologia. 2019;**51**(11):e13440

[12] Hsu CT, Lee CI, Huang CC, Wang TE, Chang HC, Chang LS, et al. Development and integration of LensHooke® R10 for automatic and standardized diagnosis for sperm DNA fragmentation. Andrology. Mar 2023:1-8. DOI: 10.1111/andr.13419. PMID: 36869577

[13] World Health Organization. WHO Laboratory Manual for the Examination and Processing of Human Semen. Geneva: World Health Organization; 2021. ISBN: 978 92 4 0030787

[14] Zhu CH, Wei Y, Zhang SM, Chen F, Li F, Dong NJ, et al. Investigation of the mechanisms leading to human sperm DNA damage based on transcriptome analysis by RNA-seq techniques. Reproductive BioMedicine Online. 2023;**46**(1):11-19

[15] Marinaro JA, Schlegel PN. Sperm DNA damage and its relevance in fertility treatment: A review of recent literature and current practice guidelines. International Journal of Molecular Sciences. 2023;**24**(2):1446

[16] Yu S, Rubin M, Geevarughese S, Pino JS, Rodriguez HF, Asghar W. Emerging technologies for home-based semen analysis. Andrology. 2018;**6**(1):10-19

[17] Yu S, Asghar W. Home-based semen analysis. In: Emerging Technologies in Biophysical Sciences: A World Scientific Reference: Volume 2: Emerging Technologies for Fertility. Chapter 7. 2023. pp. 127-141. DOI: 10.1142/9789811226106_0007

[18] Manders M, McLindon L, Schulze B, Beckmann MM, Kremer JA, Farquhar C. Timed intercourse for couples trying to conceive. Cochrane Database of Systematic Reviews. 17 Mar 2015;(3):CD011345. DOI: 10.1002/14651858.CD011345.pub2. PMID: 25775926

[19] Kandavel V, Cheong Y. Does intra-uterine insemination have a place in modern ART practice? Best Practice & Research Clinical Obstetrics & Gynaecology. 2018;**53**:3-10

[20] Ombelet W, Dhont N, Thijssen A, Bosmans E, Kruger T. Semen quality and prediction of IUI success in male subfertility: A systematic review. Reproductive Biomedicine Online. 2014;**28**(3):300-309

[21] Mahutte NG, Arici A. Failed fertilization: Is it predictable? Current Opinion in Obstetrics and Gynecology. 2003;**15**(3):211-218

[22] Esfandiari N, Javed M, Gotlieb L, Casper R. Complete failed fertilization after intracytoplasmic sperm injection-analysis of 10 years' data. International Journal of Fertility and Womens Medicine. 2005;**50**(4):187

[23] Campos G, Sciorio R, Esteves SC. Total fertilization failure after ICSI: Insights into pathophysiology, diagnosis, and management through artificial oocyte activation. Human Reproduction Update. 5 Jul 2023;**29**(4):369-394. DOI: 10.1093/humupd/dmad007. PMID: 36977357

[24] Lee SH, Lee JH, Park YS, Yang KM, Lim CK. Comparison of clinical outcomes between in vitro fertilization (IVF) and intracytoplasmic sperm injection (ICSI) in IVF-ICSI split insemination cycles. Clinical and Experimental Reproductive Medicine. 2017;**44**(2):96

[25] Malizia BA, Hacker MR, Penzias AS. Cumulative live-birth rates after in vitro fertilization. New England Journal of Medicine. 2009;**360**(3):236-243

[26] Zhu Q, Chen Q, Wang L, Lu X, Lyu Q, Wang Y, et al. Live birth rates in the first complete IVF cycle among 20 687 women using a freeze-all strategy. Human Reproduction. 2018;**33**(5):924-929

[27] Achermann AP, Pereira TA, Esteves SC. Microdissection testicular sperm extraction (micro-TESE) in men with infertility due to nonobstructive azoospermia: Summary of current literature. International Urology and Nephrology. 2021;**53**(11):2193-2210

[28] Son WY, Chung JT, Chan PT, Tan SL. Live birth after ICSI of micro-TESE–retrieved spermatozoa into In vitro–matured oocytes. Journal of andrology. 2011;**32**(1):23-25

[29] Eken A, Gulec F. Microdissection testicular sperm extraction (micro-TESE):

Predictive value of preoperative hormonal levels and pathology in non-obstructive azoospermia. The Kaohsiung journal of medical sciences. 2018;**34**(2):103-108

[30] Sciorio R, Angelaki E, Al-Azemi N, Elmardi A. One follicle, one egg, one embryo: A case-report of successful pregnancy obtained from a single oocyte collected. JBRA Assisted Reproduction. 2021;**25**(2):314

[31] Nomikos M, Kashir J, Lai FA. The role and mechanism of action of sperm PLC-zeta in mammalian fertilisation. Biochemical Journal. 2017;**474**(21):3659-3673

[32] Ebner T, Montag M, Montag M, Van der Ven K, Van der Ven H, Ebner T, et al. Live birth after artificial oocyte activation using a ready-to-use ionophore: A prospective multicentre study. Reproductive Biomedicine Online. 2015;**30**(4):359-365

[33] Niu X, Ruan Q, Witz CA, Wang W. Comparison of human oocyte activation between round-headed sperm injection followed by calcium ionophore treatment and normal sperm injection in a patient with globozoospermia. Frontiers in Endocrinology. 2020;**11**:183

[34] Ebner T, Tews G, Mayer RB, Ziehr S, Arzt W, Costamoling W, et al. Pharmacological stimulation of sperm motility in frozen and thawed testicular sperm using the dimethylxanthine theophylline. Fertility and Sterility. 2011;**96**(6):1331-1336

[35] Nordhoff V. How to select immotile but viable spermatozoa on the day of intracytoplasmic sperm injection? An Embryologist's view. Andrology. 2015;**3**(2):156-162

[36] ESHRE PGT-M Working Group, Carvalho F, Moutou C, Dimitriadou E, Dreesen J, Giménez C, et al. ESHRE PGT consortium good practice recommendations for the detection of monogenic disorders. Human Reproduction Open. 2020;**2020**(3):hoaa018

[37] Homer HA. Preimplantation genetic testing for aneuploidy (PGT-A): The biology, the technology and the clinical outcomes. Australian and New Zealand Journal of Obstetrics and Gynaecology. 2019;**59**(2):317-324

[38] Murphy LA, Seidler EA, Vaughan DA, Resetkova N, Penzias AS, Toth TL, et al. To test or not to test? A framework for counselling patients on preimplantation genetic testing for aneuploidy (PGT-A). Human Reproduction. 2019;**34**(2):268-275

[39] Penzias A, Bendikson K, Butts S, Coutifaris C, Falcone T, Fossum G, et al. The use of preimplantation genetic testing for aneuploidy (PGT-A): A committee opinion. Fertility and Sterility. 2018;**109**(3):429-436

Chapter 6

Erectile Dysfunction Caused by Cavernous Leakage

Ralf Herwig

Abstract

Erectile dysfunction (ED) is a big issue in various populations with up to 30% of young men suffering from this condition. Unfortunately, treatment schemes are currently mainly focused on elderly patients with chronic disorders. In younger patients, ED is more a vascular problem, which affects the storage capacity of the penis. The impact of penile blood supply on erectile function was recognized some 500 years ago. At the turn of the twentieth century, the first results of penile venous ligation were published. Simple isolated ligation of the deep dorsal vein in humans for ED due to venous leak is currently not recommended, due to some reported low long-term success rates. This was, as shown in several literature reports, obviously due to insufficient technical possibilities. Technical development in imaging and vascular and endovascular treatment have dramatically evolved our understanding of this underlying condition in the past 20 years and turned this disease into a long-term treatable condition. The current state-of-the-art work-up of the underlying condition, using the newest imaging technologies with color Doppler ultrasound and CT scan with additional three-dimensional reconstruction, is to show the surgeon exactly the points to focus on. Additionally, a so-called corporo-venous insufficiency can be recognized as a mainly combined condition, affecting peripheral and more proximal drainage pathways at the same time.

Keywords: erectile dysfunction, venous leak, venous leak diagnostic, venous leak treatment, CT cavernosography

1. Introduction

Erectile dysfunction (ED) is a big issue in various populations with up to 30% of young men suffering from this condition with an increasing tendency.

Cavernovenous leakage is a venous insufficiency located at the penis in which blood fails to accumulate in the corpora cavernosa because of pathological drainage of blood from the penis due to an abnormal or insufficient venous network [1, 2].

Consequently, pressure in the corpora cavernosa does not rise properly, and the resulting erection is insufficient to achieve or maintain intromission during sexual intercourse.

Furthermore, ED commonly affects the physical, psychological, and social health both of patients and their families, which can have an overall detrimental effect on the quality of life [3–5].

Papaverine intracavernosal injections (ICIs) [6] and oral medications were introduced 21 years ago [7] and have revolutionized the medical treatment of ED. Unfortunately, treatment schemes are currently mainly focused on dealing with relevant chronic disorders in elderly patients. Overall, oral treatments with PDE5 inhibitors (e.g., sildenafil (Viagra), vardenafil (Levitra), tardalafil (Cialis), and avenafil (Spedra)) are ineffective in about 30% of patients with ED [8, 9]. Despite a drug-induced increase in inflow, cavernovenous leakage is responsible for the failure to retain the blood in the penis in half of these cases [10, 11].

Up to 86% of patients resistant to intracavernous drug injection with papaverine or prostaglandin E1 have a cavernovenous leakage [12, 13].

A cavernovenous leakage is also responsible for half of the cases of severe ED, which affects 1–4% of men under the age of 25 years [14, 15].

Despite its high prevalence, cavernovenous leakage usually remains undiagnosed. Consequently, young patients with drug-resistant ED refusing a penile implant are unable to achieve sufficient and satisfying sexual intercourse.

Contrary to the long-held belief that erectile dysfunction due to venous leak is a purely human problem, there are many descriptions of this condition in different species like bulls, boars, dogs, and monkeys [16–20].

2. Pathophysiology

The etiology of venogenic erectile dysfunction is not exactly known.

Various pathologic processes were accused but none proved entirely satisfactory.

The in-flowing blood through arteries into the penis is stored in the erectile tissue, and this leads to an increase of pressure in the penis and an increase of length and hardness of the penis.

Known possible causes of the venous leak are congenital vascular anomalies, arterial insufficiency, trauma and post-priapism, diabetes, and Peyronie's disease [21].

Notwithstanding this, there are a plethora of other causes, and the exact epidemiology is not fully understood up to now.

Venous insufficiency in principle [22] can result from

1. structural changes in the vein wall (hereditary) [23],

2. venous hypertension (e.g., Peyronie's disease),

3. inflammation (e.g., diabetes),

4. alterations in shear stress, and

5. improper closure of emissary veins.

A leak will result in the outflow of blood from the penis and an insufficient erection.

1. Hereditary and acquired conditions inside the tunica albuginea or outside the cavernous corpus itself can lead to a clinically significant venous leak.

2. Cavernosal smooth muscle damage results in insufficient sinusoidal relaxation and expansion during tumescence, leading to improper closure of emissary veins as the albuginea layers are inadequately compressed.

The majority of venous leak conditions are either located outside the corpus cavernous or inside the tunica albuginea (e.g., Peyronie's disease) itself and cause a more physical problem. Therefore, the underlying physical mechanisms are further discussed in the next chapters.

The tunica albuginea of the corpora cavernosa has a bi-layered structure with multiple sublayers. The inner layer bundles are oriented circularly and support the cavernous tissue [24].

The radiating columns emanating intracavernously from this layer act like struts, enlarging the septum and providing substantial support to the erectile tissue. The outer layer bundles are oriented longitudinally. These fibers extend from the tip of the corpus cavernosum to the proximal crura, where they enter the inferior pubic ramus [24].

On a cellular level, the intracorporal pressure of patients with cavernovenous leakage is significantly lower than in healthy controls with resultant atrophy to the tunica albuginea. This in turn is resulting in a failure of compression both of the subtunical venular plexus and the emissary veins, consequently leading to a venous leak [25].

Therefore, patients' veno-occlusive dysfunction can also or additionally result from endothelial dysfunction and damage to the trabecular smooth muscle content because of ongoing multifactorial degenerative processes [21].

If any hereditary or acquired condition can lead or add to these degenerative processes of cavernous tissue, then it cannot be answered up to now.

3. Physical principles

Irrespective of many assumptions, some of which are mystical, the processes in the penis, similar to hydraulics, are also subject to the physical laws of hydrostatics and hydrodynamics.

The use of cadavers, which eliminated the influence of hormonal, arterial, neurological, sinusoidal, pharmacological, and psychological factors, demonstrates that the human erection is fundamentally a mechanical event contingent on venous competence [26].

In principle, the development of an erection can be divided into two phases:

1. Filling phase:

   A. Filling of the body of the penis via the inlet (arteries).

   B. Reduction—blocking the outlet (veins). The pressure in the cavernous corpus can reach the blood pressure (130 mmHg to 150 mmHg) at most.

2. Stiffening phase

A. Compression of the cavernous corpus on the part of the body that is surrounded by muscles (pelvic floor muscles). This increases the pressure in the penis up to 10–40 times the blood pressure to achieve a full erection. Due to the compression, the pressure propagates evenly in all directions.

B. In the event of a disturbance in the pressure on the lateral surface of the penis, there is a drop in pressure in the penis and, thus, changes in shape that affect the firmness of the penis.

Blood as a liquid shows no resistance to changes in shape but great resistance to changes in volume and is, therefore, subject to the criteria of an incompressible medium.

According to the principles of hydrostatic pressure by Pascal, this propagates evenly in all directions.

If a flowing liquid (blood) does not change its volume, the same volume of liquid must flow through the different cross sections of the line (artery, penis, and vein) every second. According to the Bernoulli equation, the sum of the pressure level, the velocity level, and the local level is constant over the entire length of the line (artery, penis, and vein). This means that the total pressure of the liquid is the same at every point.

With a "simple" blockage of the venous outflow, the pressure in the penis increases to the maximum of the blood pressure. In practice, this leads to the state of full tumescence.

Any further increase in pressure can only be achieved by either an active additional blood supply through pumping or by compressing the body from the outside (pelvic floor muscles, mainly the ischiocavernosus muscles at the penile base).

These fundamental principles can be represented in a (simplified) model for further mathematical-physical calculations (see **Figure 1**).

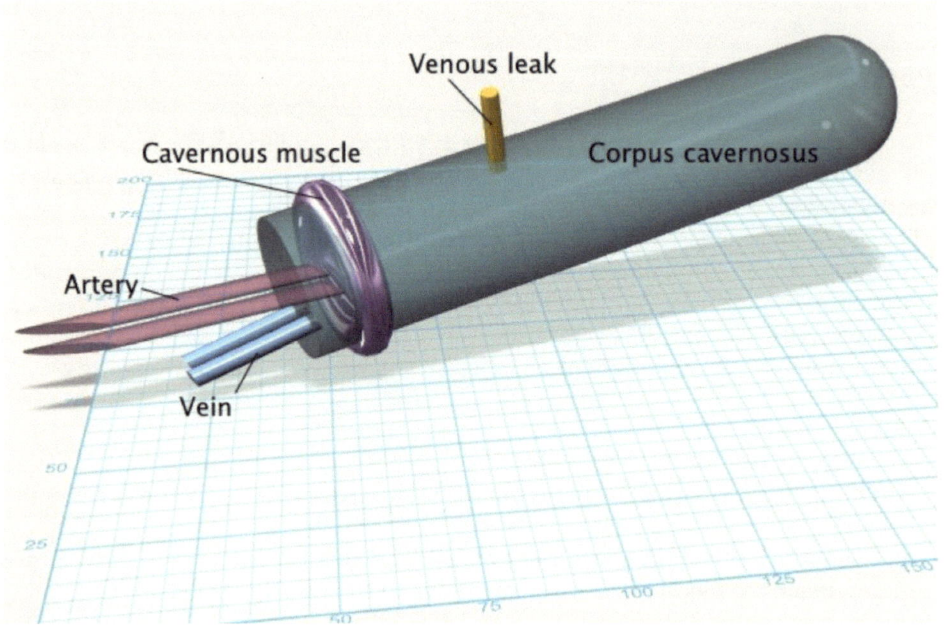

Figure 1.
Physical model of the penis.

Starting from the hydrostatics to the hydrodynamics and firmness of the penis, simple mathematical methods (finite elements) result in the spatial representation of the force and tension distributions on the surface and inside the penis. Using the physical model and the examples presented, the effluent time of the blood from the penis can be determined as a function of the total diameter of the venous leak [27].

Furthermore, prognoses can be a priori calculated in a specific patient example, which enable the surgeon to decide whether and to what extent deficiencies are likely, which are more likely to be addressed with medication or might require surgical treatment.

Application of this model demonstrates that an overall venous leak diameter of 1.5–2 mm is sufficient to induce penile de-tumescence within 30–50 s. This calculation corresponds exactly to the clinical picture (**Figure 4**).

4. Clinical presentation

Patients with congenital significant moderate-to-severe venous leak mostly report a lifelong inability to achieve a full erection under any circumstance and typically are in a younger age group [28, 29].

They usually describe erection as insufficient for intercourse or of only a short duration. Early-morning and nocturnal erections are also described as weak or absent, whereas libido is communicated as normal.

Typical complaints also include a constant soft erection barely enough for sexual intercourse, position-dependent penile rigidity, difficulty in achieving an erection, and difficulty in maintaining erections without manual stimulation. Also, a loss of penile length and girth over time and a soft glans of the penis during erection (also known as cold/floppy glans syndrome) [30, 31] are sometimes described.

Acquired cavernovenous leakage presents more or less in the same way but is preceded by a traumatic episode, for example, a road traffic accident, during sexual intercourse, or after radical prostatectomy. The patient usually offers a history of normal sexual function prior to the index accident. Not uncommonly, there may be low sexual desire secondary to the accompanying psychological burden [28].

Examination to rule out other causes of libido loss (e.g., hypogonadism) is only useful if the patient does not have normal secondary sexual characteristics, normal genitalia, or good peripheral pulses.

If a patient describes one or more of the symptoms listed above, physicians should be alert and, particularly in young patients, should look for signs that suggest an organic rather than a psychological cause of erectile dysfunction.

Such suggestive signs include

- Erectile Dysfunction persistent on all occasions where an erection is required, including with a partner or during masturbation.
- Loss of quality of morning erections.
- Loss of quality of spontaneous erections.
- Multi-treatment resistance to traditional erectile dysfunction medications including PDE5 inhibitors and ICI.

5. Diagnostic

5.1 Color Doppler Ultrasound

Dynamic color duplex Doppler ultrasound (CDDU) of the penis, first described by Lue et al. [32], is an objective and reliable diagnostic method for documenting penile hemodynamics.

Color Doppler evaluation of erectile dysfunction has also been shown to be an effective method for differentiating psychogenic and vasculogenic causes of erectile dysfunction [33].

Objective vascular testing that provides a physiologic diagnosis may help to direct the patient to an appropriate therapy.

The reasons for a lack of response to sexual stimulation based solely on medical history and standardized questionnaires (e.g., International Index of Erectile Function [IIEF] [34]) can be misleading.

Penile CDDU is required to complete evaluation in young males with primary or secondary ED and/or a history of pelvic trauma, substance abuse, prior to surgical procedures to treat Peyronie's disease. A distinction can be made between psychogenic and organic, particularly in the presence of a venous leak and in forensic cases.

The CDDU is first performed in a relaxed state, scanning the entire penis (in B-mode image) using a 7.5–12-MHz linear array ultrasound probe. This is followed by an intracorporal injection using a single or combination of vasoactive agents (e.g., prostaglandin E1, phentolamine, and papaverine), and CDDU is performed at various time points [33].

Criteria for diagnosing a venous leak are differing in various publications.

It is commonly agreed that a peak systolic blood flow (PSV) > 30 cm/s, an end-diastolic velocity (EDV) of < 3 cm/s, and a resistance index > 0.8 are generally considered normal.

A PSV below 25 cm/s is diagnostic of arterial insufficiency as the cause of ED [33, 35].

The EDV and the corresponding calculation of the resistive index (RI) are informative about penile veno-occlusion. Venogenic ED (corporo-venocclusive dysfunction or venous leak) is deemed present when the EDV and the resulting RI are abnormal with a normal PSV. Mixed vascular insufficiency is diagnosed when both PSV and EDV values were abnormal.

Using the evaluation of PSV, EDV, and RI measurements, the peak tumescence, and rigidity response, based upon the clinical history, the patient's penile vascular status can be classified as nonvascular, partial arterial, arterial, partial venous, venous, borderline mixed, or mixed as detailed in **Table 1**.

Furthermore, it is postulated that proper diagnosis of venous leakage should include both color Doppler flow analysis and computed tomography cavernosography for adequate patient selection and treatment planning [36].

5.2 Subtraction angiography and magnetic resonance tomography (MRI)

Either subtraction angiography or high-resolution arterial images similar to digital subtraction angiography with a CT scanner can be obtained [37] to demonstrate arterial inflow deficiencies.

	PSV	EDV	RI
Nonvascular	>30 cm/s	<3 cm/s	>0.8
Partial arterial	Between 25 and 30 cm/s	<3 cm/s	>0.8
Arterial	<25 cm/s	<3 cm/s	>0.8
Partial venous	30 cm/s or above	3–6 cm/s	0.6–0.8
Venous	30 cm/s or above	6 cm/s or above	<0.6
Borderline mixed	Between 25 and 30 cm/s	3–6 cm/s	0.6–0.8
Mixed	<25 cm/s	6 cm/s or above	<0.6

Table 1.
Classification of ED according to CDDU vascular status.

MRI can contribute useful information for many different pathologies in the penis. It is probably useful in investigating a painful penile implant or acute low-flow priapism. Sometimes, it may be useful for local staging of penile cancer, for localization of penile fracture, or for imaging complex cases of fibrosis.

But, in many cases, it is not convincingly superior to clinical examination or ultrasound.

Images of the venous system with an MR angiography may demonstrate the branches of the internal iliac vessels and can be used to plan pelvic revascularization, but are not of adequate resolution to show the penile vessels well, and conventional angiography is superior [38].

In evaluating erectile dysfunction, MR imaging has only limited value and has not yet proved adequately superior to other modalities to justify its routine use [39].

5.3 Three-dimensional (3D) computed tomography (CT) cavernosography

Recent technological developments allow us to reconstruct three-dimensional (3D) images from cross-sectional image data.

CT cavernosography can more accurately describe the anatomical and pathological conditions, either before or after interventions on the vascular system of the penis, than currently used plain X-ray methods. Furthermore, based on this technique, new functional and therapeutical models and principles can be developed to more effectively cure vasculogenic erectile dysfunction.

A penile CDDU only describes the presence or absence, and possibly the hemodynamic extent, of a venous leak. Therefore, this method can only tell us if there is a venous leak, not where the leak is and its complexity.

Especially in case of positive CDDU findings for venous leak, an additional CT cavernosography should be performed to morphologically demonstrate leakage of penile veins. These CT images can especially reformat data using multiplanar reconstruction, maximum intensity projection, and the volume rendering technique is able to depict details of venous leakage. This includes penile veins, the origin of the crural vein, the formation of the periprostatic venous plexus, the pudendal veins, and a pathological drainage into iliac or femoral veins.

According to this technique, penile venous leak drainage can be divided into three groups: superficial veins, intermediate veins, and deep veins [40, 41].

Hence, CT cavernosography not only is beneficial in terms of diagnosing a venous leak but is also useful for patient selection for either surgical or endovascular management.

According to Ye et al., CT cavernosography should be performed after intracavernosal injection of 20 μg prostaglandin E1. Afterward, a 7-G needle is placed into the corpora cavernosum and injection of 30–60 ml of 30% nonionic iodinated contrast medium (320 mg ml^{-1}) diluted with saline is performed using an infusion velocity of 6–180 ml min^{-1} [41]. Scanning range extends from the upper brim of the true pelvis to the most distant level of the penis. The data constructive section thickness is 1 mm with a reconstruction increment of 1 mm for post-processing.

The superior visualization of the complex venous draining system in a 3D-CT cavernosography was first described by Virag and Paul [42] and could be verified by Ye et al. [41], Uhl [43], Herwig et al. [44–46], and Xu et al. [47].

3D-CT cavernosography after ICI is able to differentiate between various venous pathways in men with venous origin ED, leading to this new anatomical classification [42].

In **Figure 2**, the 3D-CT cavernosography demonstrates no venous outflow with a completely competent closing mechanism and can be diagnosed to have no venous leak after prostaglandin E1stimulation with a venous drainage classification A according to Virag et al. [42].

The picture in **Figure 3A** and **B** describes the complexity of venous leakage disease and the need for a more combined renovation of the situation.

This might also explain the fact that neither simple ligation of only penile veins nor ligation of crural veins could deliver good long-term results in the past.

Due to the fact that the related veins are also connected via the deep pelvic vein system, these pictures might reveal the unexplained relation between erectile dysfunction and hemorrhoids [48], as well as possible erectile dysfunction after hemorrhoid sclerotherapy [49].

These pictures with new higher sophisticated techniques also demonstrate the urgent need to reexplore the pelvic and penile veinous drainage system [41].

Therefore, this in many cases underlying combination of cavernosal and crural insufficiency should be addressed in one procedure to prevent early relapse [41, 45, 50].

6. Treatment of venous leak

Currently offered treatment options like PDE5-inhibitor treatment, ICI, testosterone substitution, psychotherapy, pelvic floor training, or penile implant do in many cases not offer a sufficient solution and harbor dangers and complications:

- PDE5 inhibitors may be not sufficient in many cases (see above).
- ICI may be not sufficient and causes tissue damage with prolonged use (see above).
- Testosterone substitution may cause infertility due to dysregulation of the pituitary-gonadal axis.
- Pelvic floor training only might be successful in patients with mild symptoms [51].
- Penile implant offers a mean life expectancy of 5–10 years before replacement or removal is needed [52].

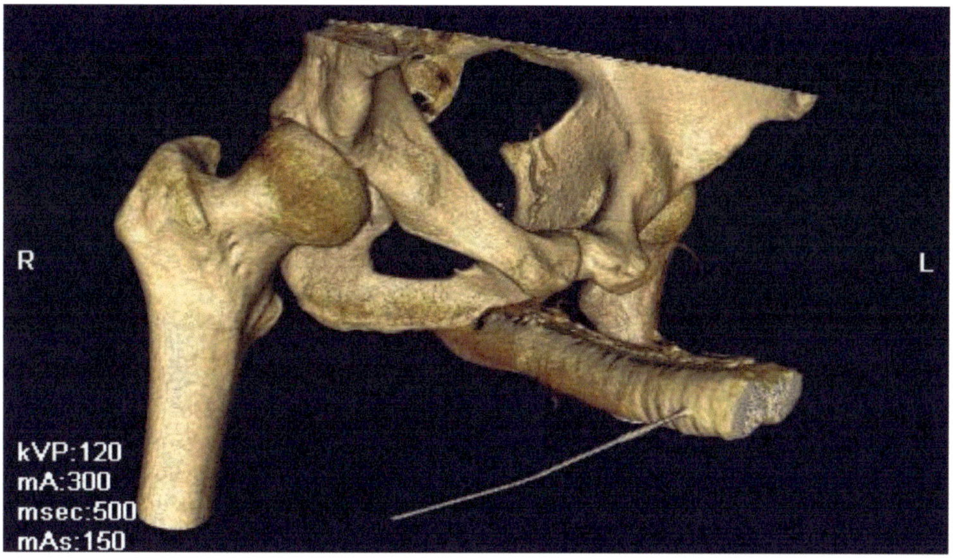

Figure 2.
No venous leak after alprostadil stimulation and venous drainage classification A according to Virag and Paul [42].

In recent studies, these aspects are respected in a newly described technique, which reaches the deep dorsal vein system, as well as the crural venous system [53–55].

The deep dorsal vein is prepared at the proximal penis shaft. A ligation of the vein toward the glans closes the primary leak from the deep dorsal vein. Furthermore, the major penile leakage points, localized by 3D-CT cavernosography, can be closed using distal and proximal ligations. In the second step, a 5F-Angiokatheter is inserted into the proximal part of the vein toward the periprostatic plexus. Under Valsalva maneuver, which must be performed by the patients, the blood flow is reduced or completely stopped in the lower pelvis equal to the compression described in general surgery guidelines for foam sclerosing of various veins.

When injecting polidocanol as a sclerosing agent during Valsalva maneuver, the agent can stay longer at the venous wall and the effect of the sclerosing therapy is maximized. In optimal cases, no residual crural or deep dorsal vein leakage can be detected after combined ligation of the deep dorsal vein and antegrade (toward the prostatic plexus) sclerotherapy procedure.

Therefore, this method is providing a therapy for deep dorsal vein and crural venous leakage in a minimal invasive setting at the same time [53–55].

With this newly described technique, at a 3-month follow-up, 77 out of 96 patients (80.21%) reported to have sufficient erections for vaginal insertion without the use of any drug or additional device [55].

These data could be verified by Carrino et al. [53], who recently reported a success rate of over 90% in more than 170 patients treated with this combined technique. Furthermore, the overall cure rate was 77%, which exceeds the effectiveness of PDE5-inhibitor therapy and additionally offers a long-term cure for erectile dysfunction [53].

More recently, Allaire et al. reported a primary success rate of 73.3% and a secondary success rate of 82.2% after a 14-month follow-up, preoperative work-up, embolization, and open surgery during the same procedure. This allowed patients

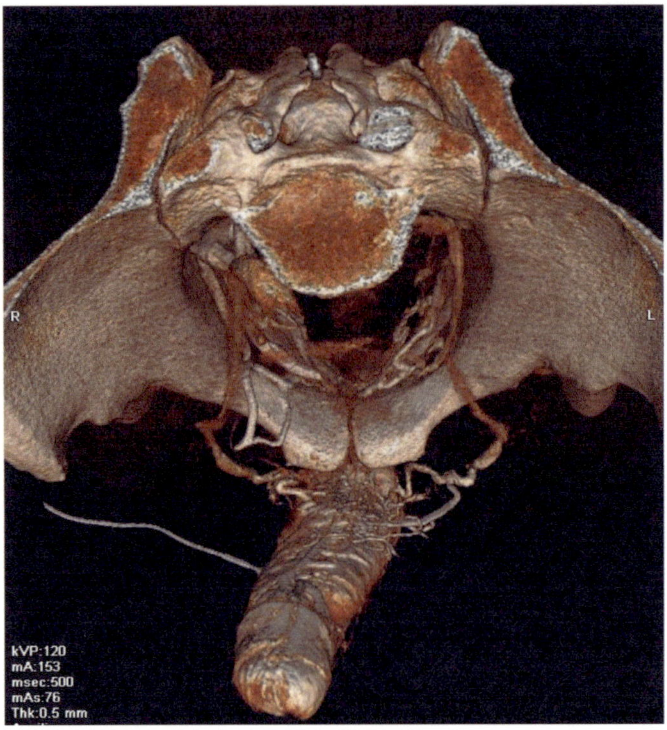

(a)

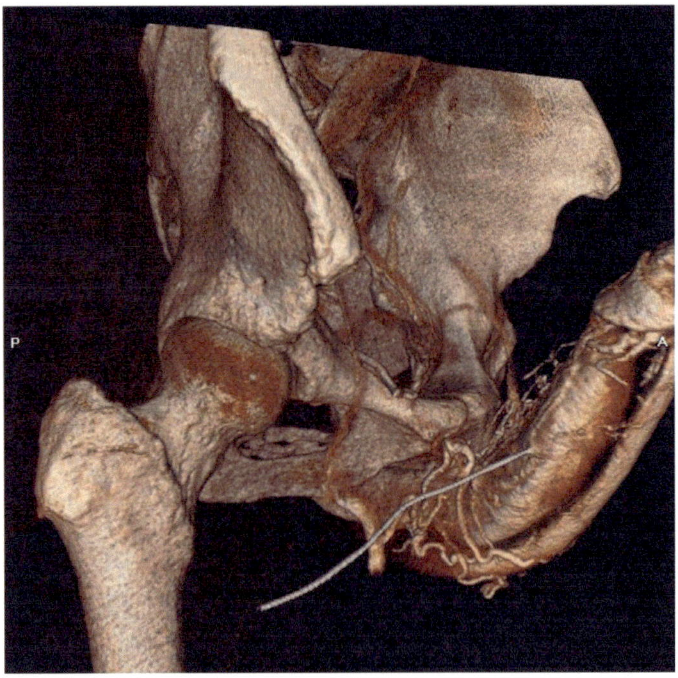

(b)

Figure 3.
(A) Venous leak Type D according to Virag and Paul [42] (view into the pelvis) and (B) venous leak Type D according to Virag and Paul [42] (view from the side).

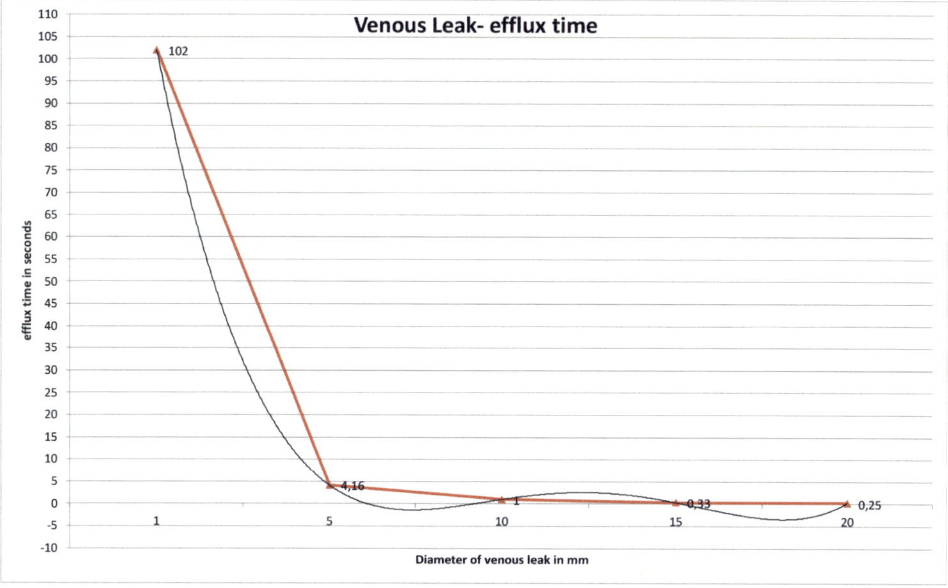

Figure 4.
Blood outflow time according to total diameter of venous leak.

with ED resistant to oral medications to achieve intercourse with normal unaided penetration [50].

In a very recent meta-analysis of almost 540 patients [46], these new and encouraging techniques demonstrated results with a short-term success rate of nearly 80% and long-term success in 73.7% of treated patients.

Regarding the applied method, a slight advantage toward a combination of ligation and antegrade sclerotherapy is found with a short-term success rate of 80% and a long-term success rate of 81.66% in altogether 267 patients [46].

According to these results with these new techniques, Rebonato et al. and Aschanbach et al. [56–58] stated that embolization techniques should be considered in all cases of erectile dysfunction due to venous leak, especially in young patients. Although the technique is not always described to be successful in restoring completely the erectile function, in most cases, the patients regain a satisfactory erectile function with additional use of small amounts of prior ineffective oral pharmacotherapy (PDE5 inhibitors) or delaying the time to penile prosthesis.

These results, although they have to be confirmed by further randomized controlled studies, verified the value of minimal invasive methods in the therapy of erectile dysfunction in patients with venous leakage. The published methods can be carried out under local anesthesia and do not contain major risks or complications [46].

A combined therapy model is possibly needed to support mostly young patients suffering from venous leak caused ED and prevent them at least partially from lifelong continuous medical treatment with all well-known disadvantages and complications.

A systematic review of the literature revealed a significant number of recent studies dealing with new minimally invasive methods that provide a potential solution for venous leakage [46].

The reported long-term results demonstrate significant improvement in ED caused by venous leakage [46].

Over 30 published studies were found in the literature with good results after minimal invasive treatment of cavernovenous leak. Altogether, 13 comparable studies including 538 patients, in which a mean short-term success rate of almost 80% and a mean long-term success rate of up to 74% were achieved (**Table 1**). None of these studies described major complications [46], it is essential to inform the patient about the possible unsuccessful result and perhaps additional treatment with low-dose PDE5 inhibitors to restore over years additionally acquired corporal smooth muscle weakness. Therefore, good patient compliance is essential.

Improvements in techniques, imaging, and sclerosing agents have opened the door for sophisticated minimally invasive venous embolization procedures [59].

Although venous surgery or embolization for the treatment of venous-occlusive disease is in general, according to some guidelines, still not recommended, these procedures can be performed with appropriate informed consent and should follow standardized methods of diagnosis as described above. The work-up before and after surgical treatment should include the use of standardized questionnaires (IIEF) and a long-term (24-month minimum) follow-up [59].

According to Sohn et al., young patients with congenital, post-inflammatory, or post-traumatic leaks may be considered for vein ligation with informed consent. The choice of treatment offered should be decided on available wisdom and infrastructure, the experience and preference of the performer, and be based on the site, nature, and size of the venous leak [60].

Besides simple surgical ligation of penile draining veins, endovascular treatment and combined focused methods may demonstrate more promising results [36].

7. Summary

Veno-occlusive dysfunction resulting in ED is undoubtedly a definite clinical entity but remains under-researched. Unfortunately, a significant number of questions at all stages of the patient pathway are unanswered up to now.

The inability to account for the brought range of degrees of arterial insufficiency and by the potential presence of minor but still significant venous leak sites under-detected in the presence of a greater leak is hindering the investigations. In many cases, the true etiology of the disease remains elusive, since the diagnostic clarification is largely standardized, but reliable reproducibility has not yet been fully achieved.

Offered management options in the past were mainly based on resection or ligation of the venous drainage either at the penis or inside the lower pelvis with a significant decline in efficacy after a follow-up exceeding 12 months, perhaps because of collateral drainage.

It is obvious that venous leakage represents a spectrum of severity. Clinically there seems to be a critical level of dysfunction, in part probably related to arterial inflow and volumetric change of the penis, at which a patient becomes symptomatic. As a result, with higher degrees of arterial insufficiency, a lower degree of veno-occlusive dysfunction would result in ED than would be required in the presence of adequate arterial inflow.

ED is an increasingly important issue, especially in young men. While current treatment strategies focus mainly on older men, young patients are more interested in a definitive or at least longer-term solution to the problem, rather than lifelong medical treatment. Various chronic disorders have been reported to be associated with elevated rates of ED including depression, diabetes, and cardiovascular and neurological disease in older men. This is mainly not the case in young men. Therefore, properly selected cases of young men may benefit from invasive treatment of cavernovenous leak treatment, and current general treatment strategies in young men should be reconsidered.

A systematic literature review demonstrates possible acceptable short-term and long-term success rates in properly selected cases, justifying a new look at the treatment of cavernovenous leak in young men. Modern techniques such as 3D-CT cavernosography may provide unprecedented opportunities for imaging and surgical planning.

Based on these data, a precise outflow blockage can be performed, not only in peripheral veins but also in deeper pelvic veins. The outcome of this technically advanced procedure is honored with an extraordinary long-term outcome of curing up to 82% of patients without further usage of additional treatment.

Author details

Ralf Herwig[1,2]

1 Heimerer-College, Pristina, Kosovo

2 German Medical Center, Dubai, United Arabic Emirates

*Address all correspondence to: dr.ralf.herwig@gmail.com

References

[1] Hsu GL, Hung YP, Tsai MH, Hsieh CH, Chen HS, Molodysky E, et al. Penile veins are the principal component in erectile rigidity: A study of penile venous stripping on defrosted human cadavers. Journal of Andrology. 2012;**33**:1176-1185

[2] Lue TF. Erectile dysfunction. The New England Journal of Medicine. 2000;**342**:1802-1813

[3] Feldman HA, Goldstein I, Hatzichristou DG, Krane RJ, McKinlay JB. Impotence and its medical and psychosocial correlates: Results of the Massachusetts Male Aging Study. The Journal of Urology. 1994;**151**:54-61

[4] Fisher WA, Eardley I, McCabe M, Sand M. Erectile dysfunction (ED) is a shared sexual concern of couples I: Couple conceptions of ED. The Journal of Sexual Medicine. 2009;**6**:2746-2760

[5] Salonia A, Castagna G, Saccà A, Ferrari M, Capitanio U, Castiglione F, et al. Is erectile dysfunction a reliable proxy of general male health status? The case for the International Index of Erectile Function-Erectile Function domain. The Journal of Sexual Medicine. 2012;**9**:2708-2715

[6] Virag R. Intracavernous injection of papaverine for erectile failure. Lancet. 1982;**2**:938

[7] Goldstein I, Lue TF, Padma-Nathan H, Rosen RC, Steers WD, Wicker PA. Oral sildenafil in the treatment of erectile dysfunction. Sildenafil Study Group. The New England Journal of Medicine. 1998;**338**:1397-1404

[8] Gong B, Ma M, Xie W, Yang X, Huang Y, Sun T, et al. Direct comparison of tadalafil with sildenafil for the treatment of erectile dysfunction: A systematic review and meta-analysis. International Urology and Nephrology. 2017;**49**:1731-1740

[9] Stuckey BG, Jadzinsky MN, Murphy LJ, Montorsi F, Kadioglu A, Fraige F, et al. Sildenafil citrate for treatment of erectile dysfunction in men with type 1 diabetes: Results of a randomized controlled trial. Diabetes Care. 2003;**26**:279-284

[10] Wespes E, Rammal A, Garbar C. Sildenafil non-responders: Haemodynamic and morphometric studies. European Urology. 2005;**48**:136-139

[11] Zhu YC, Zhao JL, Wu YG, Yuan YM, Lian WQ, Zhang J, et al. Clinical features and treatment options for Chinese patients with severe primary erectile dysfunction. Urology. 2010;**76**:387-390

[12] Fürst G, Müller-Mattheis V, Cohnen M, Trautner C, Haastert B, Saleh A, et al. Venous incompetence in erectile dysfunction: Evaluation with color-coded duplex sonography and cavernosometry/-graphy. European Radiology. 1999;**9**:35-41

[13] Rajfer J, Rosciszewski A, Mehringer M. Prevalence of corporeal venous leakage in impotent men. The Journal of Urology. 1988;**140**:69-71

[14] Ludwig W, Phillips M. Organic causes of erectile dysfunction in men under 40. Urologia Internationalis. 2014;**92**:1-6

[15] Tal R, Voelzke BB, Land S, Motarjem P, Munarriz R, Goldstein I, et al. Vasculogenic erectile dysfunction

in teenagers: A 5-year multi-institutional experience. BJU International. 2009;**103**:646-650

[16] Aboseif SR, Wetterauer U, Breza J, Benard F, Bosch R, Stief CG, et al. The effect of venous incompetence and arterial insufficiency on erectile function: An animal model. The Journal of Urology. 1990;**144**:790-793

[17] Ashdown RR, David JS, Gibbs C. Impotence in the bull: (1) Abnormal venous drainage of the corpus cavernosum penis. The Veterinary Record. 1979;**104**:423

[18] Ashdown RR, Gilanpour H, David JS, Gibbs C. Impotence in the bull: (2) occlusion of the longitudinal canals of the corpus cavernosum penis. The Veterinary Record. 1979;**104**:598-603

[19] Ashdown RR, Barnett SW, Ardalani G. Impotence in the boar 2: Clinical and anatomical studies on impotent boars. The Veterinary Record. 1982;**110**:349-356

[20] Lue TF. The mechanism of penile erection in the monkey. Seminars in Urology. 1986;**4**:217-224

[21] Montorsi F, Adaikan G, Becher E, Giuliano F, Khoury S, Lue TF, et al. Summary of the recommendations on sexual dysfunctions in men. The Journal of Sexual Medicine. 2010;**7**:3572-3588

[22] Piazza G. Varicose veins. Circulation. 2014;**130**:582-587

[23] Kaba R, Pearce I. Venous leak and erectile dysfunction–an important differential. Journal of Clinical Urology. 2020;**13**:33-39

[24] Brock G, Hsu GL, Nunes L, von Heyden B, Lue TF. The anatomy of the tunica albuginea in the normal penis and Peyronie's disease. The Journal of Urology. 1997;**157**:276-281

[25] Shafik A, Shafik I, El Sibai O, Shafik AA. On the pathogenesis of penile venous leakage: Role of the tunica albuginea. BMC Urology. 2007;**7**:14

[26] Hsu GL, Hsieh CH, Wen HS, Chen YC, Chen SC, Mok MS. Penile venous anatomy: An additional description and its clinical implication. Journal of Andrology. 2003;**24**:921-927

[27] Herwig R, Bayerl M. Superficial tunica albuginea rupture as initial starting point of Peyronie's disease: A topic for interdisciplinary consideration. BioMed Research International. 2015;**2015**:751372

[28] Reed-Maldonado AB, Lue TF. A syndrome of erectile dysfunction in young men. Translational Andrology and Urology. 2016;**5**:228-234

[29] Chen SC, Hsieh CH, Hsu GL, Wang CJ, Wen HS, Ling PY, et al. The progression of the penile vein: Could it be recurrent. Journal of Andrology. 2005;**26**:53-60

[30] Bickell M, Manimala N, Parker J, Steixner B, Wiegand L, Carrion R. Floppy Glans syndrome: Pathogenesis and treatment. Sex Medical Review. 2016;**4**:149-156

[31] Schramek P, Waldhauser M. Isolated glans insufficiency due to venous leakage. Urology. 1990;**35**:307-309

[32] Lue TF, Hricak H, Marich KW, Tanagho EA. Vasculogenic impotence evaluated by high-resolution ultrasonography and pulsed Doppler spectrum analysis. Radiology. 1985;**155**:777-781

[33] Sikka SC, Hellstrom WJ, Brock G, Morales AM. Standardization of vascular

assessment of erectile dysfunction: Standard operating procedures for duplex ultrasound. The Journal of Sexual Medicine. 2013;**10**:120-129

[34] Rosen RC, Riley A, Wagner G, Urology IHO. The international index of erectile function (IIEF): A multidimensional scale for assessment of erectile dysfunction. Urology. 1997;**49**:822

[35] Hatzimouratidis, K., F. Giuliano, I. Moncada, A. Muneer, A. Salonia, and P. Verze. EAU Guidelines on Erectile Dysfunction, Premature Ejaculation, Penile Curvature and Priapism. Available from: https://d56bochluxqnz.cloudfront.net/media/EAU-Guidelines-on-Male-Sexual-Dysfunction-2019.pdf

[36] Hoppe H, Diehm N. Venogenic erectile dysfunction: Diagnosis on computed tomography cavernosography and endovascular treatment using an anterograde access via deep dorsal penile vein. CVIR Endovascular. 2022;**5**:10

[37] Kawanishi Y, Lee KS, Kimura K, Kojima K, Yamamoto A, Numata A. Feasibility of multi-slice computed tomography in the diagnosis of arteriogenic erectile dysfunction. BJU International. 2001;**88**:390-395

[38] Kirkham A. MRI of the penis. British Journal of Radiology. 2012;**85**:86-93

[39] Kirkham AP, Illing RO, Minhas S, Minhas S, Allen C. MR imaging of nonmalignant penile lesions. Radiographics. 2008;**28**:837-853

[40] Gratzke C, Angulo J, Chitaley K, Dai YT, Kim NN, Paick JS, et al. Anatomy, physiology, and pathophysiology of erectile dysfunction. The Journal of Sexual Medicine. 2010;**7**:445-475

[41] Ye T, Li J, Li L, Yang L. Computed tomography cavernosography combined with volume rendering to observe venous leakage in young patients with erectile dysfunction. The British Journal of Radiology. 2018;**91**:20180118

[42] Virag R, Paul JF. New classification of anomalous venous drainage using caverno-computed tomography in men with erectile dysfunction. The Journal of Sexual Medicine. 2011;**8**:1439-1444

[43] Uhl JF. Three-dimensional modelling of the venous system by direct multislice helical computed tomography venography: Technique, indications and results. Phlebology. 2012;**27**:270-288

[44] Herwig R, Weibl P. CT cavernosography and penile venous leak. European Urology Supplements. 2017;**16**:e2827

[45] Herwig R, Greilberger J, Weibl P. CT cavernosography and penile venous leak. JOJ Urology and Nephrology. 2017;**3**:1-5

[46] Herwig R, Kamel A, Shabsigh R. CT Cavernosography and penile venous leak therapy. Journal of Men's Health. 2019;**15**(2):12-19

[47] Xu CC, Pan YN, Tang YF, Zhang J, Wang GY, Huang QL. Comprehensive assessment of cavernosography with 320-row dynamic volume CT versus conventional cavernosography in erectile dysfunction patients caused by venous leakage. Bioscience Report. 2017;**37**(3):1-9

[48] Keller JJ, Lin HC. Haemorrhoids are associated with erectile dysfunction: A population-based study. International Journal of Andrology. 2012;**35**:867-872

[49] Pilkington SA, Bateman AC, Wombwell S, Miller R. Anatomical basis for impotence following haemorrhoid sclerotherapy. Annals of the Royal College of Surgeons of England. 2000;**82**:303-306

[50] Allaire E, Sussman H, Zugail AS, Hauet P, Floresco J, Virag R. Erectile dysfunction resistant to medical treatment caused by cavernovenous leakage: An innovative surgical approach combining pre-operative work up, embolisation, and open surgery. European Journal of Vascular and Endovascular Surgery. 2021;**61**:510-517

[51] Claes H, Baert L. Pelvic floor exercise versus surgery in the treatment of impotence. British Journal of Urology. 1993;**71**:52-57

[52] Chierigo F, Capogrosso P, Dehò F, Pozzi E, Schifano N, Belladelli F, et al. Long-term follow-up after penile prosthesis implantation-survival and quality of life outcomes. The Journal of Sexual Medicine. 2019;**16**:1827-1833

[53] Carrino M et al. Embolization of the deep dorsal vein using aethoxysklerol in the treatment of erectole dysfunction resulting from venous leakage. In: XXIII Congresso Nationale Auro.it. 2016

[54] Herwig R, Margreiter M, Kuehhas F. PELVIC venoablation for the treatment of erectile dysfunction caused by venous leakage. European Urology Supplements. 2012;**11**:87

[55] Herwig R, Sansalone S. Venous leakage treatment revisited: Pelvic venoablation using aethoxysclerol under air block technique and Valsalva maneuver. Archivio Italiano di Urologia, Andrologia. 2015;**87**:1-4

[56] Aschenbach R, Steiner T, Kerl MJ, Zangos S, Basche S, Vogl TJ. Endovascular embolisation therapy in men with erectile impotence due to veno-occlusive dysfunction. European Journal of Radiology. 2013;**82**:504-507

[57] Rebonato A, Auci A, Sanguinetti F, Maiettini D, Rossi M, Brunese L, et al. Embolization of the periprostatic venous plexus for erectile dysfunction resulting from venous leakage. Journal of Vascular and Interventional Radiology. 2014;**25**:866-872

[58] Rebonato A, Maiettini D, Ceccherini C, Nuti A, Sanguinetti F. Endovascular treatment of recurrent erectile dysfunction due to venous occlusive disease. Asian Journal of Andrology. 2017;**19**:509-510

[59] Trost LW, Munarriz R, Wang R, Morey A, Levine L. External mechanical devices and vascular surgery for erectile dysfunction. The Journal of Sexual Medicine. 2016;**13**:1579-1617

[60] Sohn M, Hatzinger M, Goldstein I, Krishnamurti S. Standard operating procedures for vascular surgery in erectile dysfunction: Revascularization and venous procedures. The Journal of Sexual Medicine. 2013;**10**:172-179

Chapter 7

Libido Boosting Functional Foods

Neelesh Kumar Maurya

Abstract

Libido is a sexual desire or drive. Libido is biological desire's emotional energy, especially sexual desire. Biopsychosocial variables affect libido. Biologically, sex hormones and nucleus accumbent neurotransmitters (mainly testosterone and dopamine) govern human desire. Working, family, mentality, and stress might affect libido. Medical disorders, drugs, lifestyle, relationships, and age might affect libido (e.g., puberty). Hypersexuality is having frequent or suddenly increased sexual impulses; hyposexuality is the opposite. In psychoanalytic thought, libido is a mental drive or energy, connected with sexual instinct but is also present in other innate urges. A man may want sex but not be able to act on it, or may not for medical, moral, or religious reasons. Repressing or sublimating an urge is psychological. One can participate in sexual activity without a sire. Stress, illness, and pregnancy affect sperm drive. Testosterone, estrogen, progesterone, oxytocin, and norepinephrine act as serotonin This book chapter talks about how functional foods such as spinach, dark chocolate, peppers, green tea, oysters, crab, and pumpkin seeds, which contain neurotransmitters, affect libido.

Keywords: libido, sex, neurotransmitters, functional foods, sea foods

1. Introduction

Libido is a general sexual urge or drive. Libido is influenced by biopsychosocial factors. Human desire is governed biologically by sex hormones and nucleus-accumbent neurotransmitters (primarily testosterone and dopamine) [1–3]. Work, family, mensuration, and stress can all have an impact on libido. Medical conditions, drugs, lifestyle, internal issues, and age (puberty) can all have an impact on libido. When a man has frequent or unexpectedly increased sexual impulses, this is referred to as hypersexuality [4]. The inverse is hyposexuality. Libido is defined by psychoanalytic theory as a mental drive or energy associated with sexual instincts and other instinctual urges and drives. For men, a man may desire sex but be unable to act on it for medical, moral, or religious reasons [5]. It is psychological to suppress or sublimate an urge. Sexual activity can be performed without the presence of desire. Stress, illness, and pregnancy can all have an impact on sex drive [6, 7]. According to van Anders et al. '*2022* study, men desire sex more than women. Sexual impulses are typically essential in the formation and maintenance of internal relationships. Sexual disinterest can harm relationships [7]. Changes in a partner's sexual desires can cause relationship problems if left unresolved. Infidelity may indicate that a partner's changing sexual demands are unsatisfactory in the current relationship. Problems may arise because of disparate sexual impulses or poor communication. There is no universally accepted measure of healthy desexualization. Others prefer to have sex only once a year or never at all. Someone who has not been sexually active for an extended period may have a hypoactive sexual drive or be asexual. Sigmund Freud, the term's originator, defined libido as "the energy, seen as a quantitative magnitude of all "love" instincts." Sigmund Freud referred to it as the id, the unconscious structure of the psyche. He compared it to hunger, the desire for power, and so on, claiming that it is an essential human instinct [8]. Freud proposed a series of developmental stages in which the libido fixates on different erogenous zones, beginning with the oral stage (exemplified by an infant's pleasure in nursing), then the anal stage, the phallic stage, a latency stage, and finally the genital stage at puberty. Karl Abraham later added the subdivisions "oral" and "anal. Sigmund Freud observed that libidinal desires can clash with superego-represent civilized behavior [9, 10]. This need to conform to society and control one's libido causes stress and disruption in the individual, prompting defeasances to disperse the psychic energy of these unfulfilled, primarily unconscious needs. Overuse of ego defenses leads to neurosis. Psychoanalysis seeks to bring id desires into consciousness so that they can be addressed directly, thereby removing ego defenses. Desire, according to Freud, evolves. Failure to adjust to these various stages can result in libidinal energy becoming "damped up" or fixated on them, resulting in pathological character traits in maturity. Psychopaths, according to Freud, are immature. Psychoanalysis sought to bring men's fixations to their attention so that libido energy could be used constructively [8]. In psychoanalysis, Jung defined libido as psychic energy, not just sexual desire. Libido, according to Jung, is an uncontrolled desire or drive, moral or otherwise. Libido is natural hunger. From a genetic standpoint, libido is made up of biological needs such as food, thirst, sleep, and sex, as well as emotional states or effects. Duality (opposition) fosters the psyche's energy (or libido), which Jung claims can only be expressed symbolically. Psychoanalysis may reveal these symbols as "fantasy images" that embody the formless contents of the libido. A psychological craving, movement, displacement, or structure is defined as a desire [9, 10].

2. Factors that influence libido

2.1 Endogenous substance

Dopaminergic action in the mesolimbic pathway is principally responsible for libido regulation (ventral tegmental area and nucleus accumbent). Because of this, dopamine and other related trace amines (most notably phenethylamine) that influence dopamine neurotransmission play an essential part in the process of controlling the desire. Other neurotransmitters, neuropeptides, and sex hormones can affect sex drive by altering the way this route functions or by acting on it directly. These include the following [1, 8, 11]:

- Testosterone (in a direct causal relationship)-in addition to several androgens
- Estrogen is (in close connection with) the female reproductive hormone.
- Progesterone (relationship)

- Oxytocin (directly correlated)
- Serotonin (the opposite of associated)
- The link between norepinephrine and
- Acetylcholine

2.2 Hormones and the menstrual cycle

Many women reports increased sexual desire in the days preceding ovulation, a woman's prime reproductive time. This cycle is influenced by menstrual testosterone levels. According to Gurian et al., testosterone affects women's sex [12]. A woman's desire for sex increases from the 24th day of her cycle until ovulation on the 14th. Testosterone levels peak on the day Women have less sexual desire and lower testosterone levels after ovulation. After ovulation, progesterone levels rise, making orgasm difficult [12, 13]. A woman's testosterone level remains constant in the latter days of her menstrual cycle, but her uterine lining increases, activating nerve endings and making her stimulated. Natural lubrication is reduced when estrogen levels are low. According to experts, menopause diminishes women's sexual desire. Menopause lowers estrogen levels, which inhibits sexual interest and causes vaginal dryness. Testosterone levels rise during menopause, which may increase desire [2, 13, 14].

2.3 Variables in sociopsychology

Sexual desire may be reduced by psychiatric or social disorders. Insecurity, tension, exhaustion, distraction, and despair are some examples. Loud noises or bright lights may impair libido. Some reasons include sexual assault, trauma, neglect, and body image difficulties. PTSD diminishes sexual desire. Patients suffering from PTSD lack trust and joy. PTSD causes sexual desire to be inhibited by vulnerability, fury, anger, and emotional shutdowns. Sexual dysfunction can impair the sex drive of trauma victims. Women's sexual drive is restored after the treatment [15]. Depression and libido loss frequently coexist, as depression reduces sex drive. Libido declines more than other symptoms in those suffering from depression [4, 6].

2.4 Physical aspects

Libido may be affected by hypothyroidism, flutamide, and a partner's beauty and fitness. Women's libido is reduced by menstrual anemia. Tobacco, alcohol, and narcotics all suppress libido. Experts believe that exercising, stopping smoking, and reducing alcohol use can increase sexual desire [16].

2.5 Medications

Anaphrodisiacs reduce libido. Psychostimulants and aphrodisiacs increase libido. It lowers libido. Isotretinoin, SSRIs, antidepressants, antipsychotics, opioids, and beta-blockers cause it. Isotretinoin and many SSRIs can impair libido and sexual function. All antidepressants reduce libido, except Wellbutrin, Desyrel, and Serzone. Prozac, Paxil, Luvox, Celexa, and Sertraline reduce libido (Zoloft). Antidepressant users reduce doses to maintain their sex drive. Others seek help for a depressed libido. Numerous individuals believe this therapy does not affect sexual desire. Testosterone regulates libido. Research shows (SHBG) that oral contraceptives reduce female libido by increasing sex hormone-binding globulin levels. SHBG inhibits testosterone. SHBG levels remain high after hormonal contraception is stopped, and no data predicts when they will decline. Oral contraceptives reduce testosterone and libido. Oral contraceptives are libido neutral. Most oral contraceptive users report consistent libido. Aging affects Male sex drives peak in their teens, while females peak in their 30s. Puberty causes a strong sex urge for 15–16 years. Female libido peaks in the mid-30s. Testosterone and estrogen affect libido. Some 10–12-year-olds are romantic or sexual. It is less romantic than desire and attraction. 25% of 11–12-year-olds "had sex thoughts." 13–14-year-old boys had more sexual urges than girls. At this age, boys are more sexual [17]. In teens, in their 20s and 30s, masturbation increases. Less than 10% of males masturbate by 10, 50% by 11–12, and most by 13–14. 20% of 13–14-year-old girls masturbate. By the mid-70s, sex desire may have decided to drop. Health, the environment, and society affect an aaginglibido [18]. Women in their 40s and 50s are more sexually active and willing to please. Family, health, connection, and well-being suppress women's sexual urges. Aging people are sexier, less responsible, and more confident. Negative people mention health. Seniors have trouble discussing their sexuality with caregivers and doctors due to age-related preconceptions. Non-western countries believe older women have lower libidos, discouraging sexuality. Pensions diminish libido. These homes discourage sex. Insecurity and gender injustice diminish desire. Seniors benefit from sex excitement, good health, sexual self-esteem, and a loving relationship.

2.6 Sexual reliance

More women than men have asexual desire disorders. Women's sexual desires are less frequent and intense than men's [19]. Lack of sexual desire can cause erectile dysfunction, but the two are different. Large doses of amphetamine or methamphetamine can cause erectile dysfunction and boost libido [20, 21]. Men's libidos can also decline with age. Several million women have a female sexual arousal disorder, but arousal is not synonymous with desire, so this finding is limited to libido. Hormonal problems, like a lack of luteinizing hormone or androgenic hormones, may cause low libido, but these ideas aren't agreed upon [22].

3. The causes of desire loss

Lack of quality sleep, high stress, poor diet, poor physical health, medications and birth control pills, low physical activity, unresolved conflicts, repressed emotions, depression, and anxiety, past sexual abuse, poor self-image and lack of self-confidence, infidelity, and menopause (or other hormonal imbalances like low thyroid) are the main psychological and emotional causes of low sex drive in men and women. Sex drives are linked to the reproductive system, but no system operates independently. If men are experiencing low sex drive, start with these main culprits and see if they can find the root cause [22].

3.1 The invisible cause of libido loss

Experts say that hidden hostility or repressed anger towards the partner can cause a lack of sex drive. Often, when a woman blames her hormones for her lack of desire, a closer look at the relationship reveals stresses, strains, and repressed anger. If a woman is fed up because her man is not romantic, never takes her out, never thanks her, or always expects her to handle contraception, it's not surprising she does not want to make love to him. Her desire wanes. Addressing these problems is harder than saying "it's all hormones." Unfortunately, it's the relationship that needs changing, not hormones. Many couples see doctors because they believe hormonal issues are causing their unhappiness. After counseling and digging deeper into the problem, it's common to find that the woman lost interest in sex due to an interior flaw in the relationship. Perhaps the man is too controlling for her. Sometimes Couples therapy can put a relationship back on track, especially if both the man and the woman can accept that the sexual problem is rooted in the relationship [23, 24].

Sometimes one or both partners refuse to face the truth that there is no magic pill to cure their problems and that they need to change their relationship—and they stop going to therapy. A woman may struggle with a lack of desire at certain times in her life. After birth, abortion, miscarriage, premenstrual tension, menopause, etc. All of these are "normal" times for women to lose sexual desire.

3.2 The role of infidelity in libido loss

Unfaithfulness can cause a loss of libido. Infidelity may be caused by a lack of libido in some cases, but it's usually a lack of intimacy. Passion is one of many elements of a relationship. Other factors that can improve sexual relations are intimacy, communication, and non-sexual contact. For women, it's not what happens now but the sum of non-sexual moments in a relationship that matters [11, 16].

3.3 Intimacy

Intimacy is the emotional, sexual, and spiritual glue that binds two people. This bond can be affected if partners do not feel connected and communicate their needs [19]. Directing more energy to outside things like a job, children, friends, or coworkers may cause this bond to dissolve. Balance must be maintained; if not, a partner may seek to get their needs met elsewhere by emotionally reconnecting with another man, which can lead to an affair. Both people in a relationship are responsible for keeping it going, so pay attention to what the partner needs from the spouse [20–22].

3.4 Multiple sex partners before marriage increase infidelity

Any sexual activity releases energy and hormones that keep couples together and build trust. When people have many casual sex partners before marriage and they end up having children, it weakens natural bonding [21]. This can cause loss, betrayal, unwanted memories, and other problems in a marriage. Having more than one sexual partner before getting married makes men more likely to be depressed, cheat on their partner, and get a divorce. This is because the power of the natural bonding agents is weakened [23].

3.5 Boredom

In "Flirting with Disaster," Samantha Cleaver writes that unchallenged partners tend to cheat more often. "The desire for growth and self-expansion can lead to unfaithfulness in a spouse" [20]. Couples should communicate their growth goals, set them, and help each other achieve them. Take classes, book weekend trips, or try a new fitness activity.

Men may be surprised by how much men's desire and intimacy grow and how this affects their sex drive. Men either grow together or grow apart; nothing stands still [23].

4. Supplements that boost sexual desire

4.1 Micronutrient supplements

Vitamin C increases genital blood flow. It removes toxins, boosts the immune system, and treats allergies naturally. Vitamin C improves the immune system and reproductive organ function. It's best to take vitamin C steadily throughout the day to maximize absorption and benefit. Overdosing more than 2000 mg daily may cause diarrhea. Chilies, guava, parsley, kiwi, broccoli, Brussel sprouts, papaya, strawberry, citrus (like oranges, grapefruit, and lemons), cantaloupe, garlic, raspberry, passion fruit, and spinach are high [25].

4.1.1 Vitamin

Vitamin E has surprising benefits. Vitamin E helps produce sex-empowering hormones for a healthy desire. It's established a mood and desire. 15 mg per day is the recommended daily allowance. As a fat-soluble vitamin, Vitamin E will stay in a man's body longer than Vitamin C, but he should not take too much. Most food sources are safe. Avocados, nuts, seeds, green leafy vegetables, fortified cereals, vegetables, grape seeds, and canola oil are natural vitamin E sources [26].

Vitamin A keeps skin, teeth, bones, vision, and urinary and vaginal linings healthy. It regulates men's immune systems to keep men healthy. Daily vitamin A intake should not exceed 7500 mcg. Cantaloupe, pink grapefruit, apricots, carrots, pumpkin, sweet potatoes, squash, broccoli, spinach, and dark leafy greens [27]. Vitamin C is a powerful antioxidant and is a must-take for any woman going through menopause. Vitamin C will help with dry, itchy skin, fatigue, osteoporosis, bloating, g and depression [25]. Vitamin D is important for women to take even before they reach menopause. They work in conjunction to keep the bones strong, which will help to stave off osteoporosis [28]. Vitamin B6: If men are having menopausal sleeping issues, this vitamin can help. It will work in the body to assist in producing serotonin 50–200 mg/day [29, 30]. Vitamin B3 is being looked at to help the level of hormones in the body during menopause [31]. Vitamin B1 and B12 can help with menopausal symptoms like moodiness, lethargy, and depression [31–33].

4.1.2 Calcium, iron, magnesium

Meats contain amino acids, zinc, and iron for sexual performance. It increases sex sensitivity by boosting brain chemicals. Look for grass-fed beef, free-range eggs, grass-fed dairy, grass-fed beef, free-range turkey, grass-fed beef liver, wild tuna, wild salmon, and buffalo [33].

4.2 Fish oil/omega- 3

This boosts brain oxygen, dopamine, and serotonin. This increases testosterone and sexual desire. These chemicals reduce anxiety and stress, which lower libido in men and women. "A lack of fatty acids can lower hormone levels and sexual desire.

Flaxseed and low-mercury fish like salmon, herring, mackerel, tuna, and halibut are natural Omega 3 sources [34].

4.3 L-Arginine

L-Arginine is great for rock-hard erections and increased ejaculate volume. If men want to boost performance, take 500 mg daily and 1000 mg before intercourse. Use with caution and discontinue if any side effects occur [34].

4.4 Glutathione

There are several nutrients that, when it comes to men's health, can help boost men's memory, performance, and sex drive. Some of these nutrients have even been shown to raise a man's body's production of testosterone, which is a particularly desirable effect [35]. According to the findings of several studies, erectile dysfunction is more common in males whose glutathione levels are low. Taking pills that boost this natural antioxidant could help with erectile dysfunction or even stop it from happening [34].

5. Herbs for an extra boost

5.1 Bee pollen

Both men and women can benefit from using bee pollen as a dietary supplement because it has been shown to increase levels of energy. It has a high concentration of enzymes, amino acids, vitamins, and minerals. Taking it will assist in enhancing sexual stamina, giving men more frequent erections, and also increasing the volume of ejaculate that they produce. Bee pollen can be purchased in a variety of formats, including tablets, capsules, and even in its living state. If Meccano locates the live freeze-dried forms in a men's health food store, they should purchase these forms because they are the most powerful [36].

5.2 Black cohosh (*Actaea racemose*)

Black cohosh has a plant-based estrogen that helps regulate hormones, bringing comfort to a wide spectrum of women suffering from menopause symptoms such as vaginal dryness, itching, moodiness, depression, and hot flashes. Black cohosh includes a plant-based estrogen that helps regulate hormones [37].

5.3 Yam (*Dioscorea alata*)

The use of wild yam as a natural menopause treatment is beneficial for maintaining healthy hormone levels, particularly progesterone. Depression, moodiness, low libido, irritability, and anger are all conditions that can be helped by taking this hormone, which also plays a function in managing moods and is used to treat these conditions [37].

5.4 Ginseng (*Panax quinquefolius*)

For thousands of years, the Chinese have utilized ginseng for the treatment of a variety of health ailments and issues, including menopause. A woman can develop an aversion to sexual activity and lose interest in it if someone has a dry vagina, even though the condition itself does not necessarily indicate a decline in her desire to have sexual encounters [37]. Ginseng is very helpful in maintaining the suppleness, moisture, and overall health of the vaginal walls, thus minimizing dryness, tearing, and pain. Ginseng is a tonic herb. Ginseng has been shown to be iseatment of sleeplessness, irritability, and hot flashes. 5% ginsenosides or 100 mg of 10% saponin ginsenosides per day, with 4–6 Lachesis of high-quality root per day [38].

5.5 Lachesis

Lachesis is an excellent choice for women who suffer from intense hot flashes during the day as well as at night. It's possible that the temperature will be even higher at night compared to during the day. There is a possibility of headaches and migraines on the left side. The woman who needs Lachesis has a propensity to be on the hotter side all the time and may have an insatiable desire for alcoholic beverages [39].

5.6 Red clover (*Trifolium pratense*)

Red Clover can help with hot flashes and mood swings. Furthermore, it is ideal to begin taking it while still experiencing PMS symptoms. In a man's physique, red clover treats a variety of female-related ailments [40].

5.7 *Ginkgo biloba*

Adults use 60–240 mg of ginkgo daily for up to 6 months. Dosages vary by formulation. Most researched products contain ginkgo leaf extracts. *G. biloba* boosts sex drive in perimenopausal and menopausal women. It helps balance hormones, boosting menopausal estrogen levels. This can boost libido and sexual desire. Ginkgo activates Leydig cells in the testes to boost testosterone and maintain cortisol levels in line, which supports healthy testosterone levels. Ginkgo boosts nitric oxide, which is needed to produce testosterone [37].

5.8 *Panax ginseng*

P. ginseng is used to treat anxiety, athletic/physical stamina, cognitive function, depression, male fertility, migraines, immunostimulants, menopausal hot flashes, and impotence. Both American and Asian ginseng can boost energy, lower blood sugar and cholesterol, reduce stress, induce relaxation, treat diabetes, and control sexual dysfunction in men. The libido-boosting properties of *P. ginseng* may stem from its stress-relieving properties. Ginseng may help with infertility by improving sexual performance, sperm count, and quality [37, 40].

5.9 Yohimbine

The increase in sexual desire caused by yohimbine does not appear to be related to testosterone. However, one human study found a weak association with free testosterone. For centuries, the bark has been used as an aphrodisiac. Yohimbe is used to treat erectile dysfunction, improve athletic performance, and lose weight, angina, high blood pressure, and diabetic neuropathy [37].

5.10 Celery

Celery increases the male aphrodisiac pheromone and androsterone. Celery can expand blood vessels, improve sex drive, and enhance climax. Celery has the sex hormone estrone, which was used to stimulate libido in ancient times. Celery was a classic appetite and sexual power stimulant. Red celery juice extract promotes bowel movement and menstrual flow. Celery is a lust actuator, which increases menstrual flow and triggers abortion in pregnant and breastfeeding women [41].

5.11 Pumpkin (*Cucurbita moschata*) seeds

According to Chinese medicine, pumpkin seeds are excellent and have antidepressant properties. Eating pumpkin seeds can affect the health of a man's prostate, which is essential for male sexual health. It improves the functioning of the prostate gland as well as the hormones in males. Myosin is essential for the contraction of muscles, and pumpkin seeds are a good source of it [42].

5.12 Bananas (*Musa acuminata*)

Potassium and riboflavin, the essential nutrients found in bananas, are known to improve libido in addition to assisting in the creation of testosterone, which is a male sex hormone [37]. Bananas include a substance called tryptophan, which contributes to an increase in the production of serotonin. Serotonin is a hormone that improves a man's mood and raises his sexual desire. Bananas contain an enzyme called bromelain that can improve impotence in men and improve their desire to have sexual encounters [42].

5.13 Walnuts (*Juglans* spp.)

The results of the study led the study's authors to the conclusion that incorporating walnuts, hazelnuts, and almonds into an unhealthy western diet may increase sexual desire (libido), as well as an improvement in the quality or intensity of orgasms. Walnuts are an excellent source of omega-3 fatty acids, which are heart-healthy fats that increase dopamine levels. Walnuts are also a good source of arginine, which is an amino acid that stimulates the body's production of nitric oxide, which in turn relaxes blood vessels and boosts circulation [43].

5.14 Avocado (*Asparagus officinalis*)

Avocado's high levels of folic acid aid in the metabolization of proteins, which gives men more energy. Avocado is a versatile culinary delight. They contain vitamin E, which is beneficial to the nails and skin. Avocados are high in vitamin B6, potassium, and monounsaturated fats [26, 37]. These promote healthy circulation and a strong heart, both of which are required for sex. Avocados naturally protect the arteries. Erectile dysfunction is more common in men with heart disease. Avocado consumption lowers the risk of metabolic syndrome, which is a risk factor for erectile dysfunction. Men with metabolic syndrome are twice as likely as women to develop ED. Avocados are versatile and easy to prepare. For breakfast, try mashed avocado on toast, or in a sandwich or salad [44].

5.15 Asparagus (*A. officinalis*)

A typical grocery store veggie is a potent aphrodisiac. Asparagus boosts libido and sexual wellness for men and women. Asparagus boosts libido. It contains B6 and folate. These minerals help with sexual health. Asparagus contains potassium, which helps produce sex hormones. Eating asparagus can improve orgasms and sexual health by increasing excitement [45].

5.16 Basil (*Ocimum basilicum*)

Studies have shown that basil can boost female fertility as well as men's desire to have sexual encounters. Some claims inhaling the aroma of basil can be beneficial for relieving headaches. Researchers mentioned that the ability to enhance blood circulation. It also talks about how basil warms the body and how this makes women more sexually attracted to each other [45].

5.17 Honey

Honey plays a crucial role in maintaining sexual health. Because it's full of natural sugars, it gives people more stamina and makes it possible to stay in bed for longer. Honey also has boron, a mineral that has been shown to have the ability to control both hormone levels and nitric oxide production. This vasodilator is released into the bloodstream during sexual excitement, and its role is to widen blood vessels. In other words, it causes the blood vessels to become more expansive [46].

5.18 Watermelon (*Citrullus lanatus*)

Citrulline is an amino acid that can be transformed into arginine, which can then be converted to nitric oxide. There is a significant amount of citrulline found in watermelons. There is some evidence that watermelons contain citrulline as well. The participants in a study that was conducted in 2007 were given 1560 g of watermelon juice daily for a period of 3 weeks, which resulted in increased levels of arginine. It is always necessary to remember that whenever drinking or extracting juice from the pulp of a watermelon, the rind of the watermelon should be included, as this is where the largest portion of citrulline is found [43].

5.19 Dark chocolate (*Cocoa*)

Cacao is a superfood, and modern foodies know it. It's antioxidant-richer than green tea or red wine. It contains phenylethylamine, which enhances excitement and well-being. The Journal of Sexual Medicine discovered that women who ate dark chocolate every day had more active sex lives than those who did not [37, 43].

5.20 Nutmeg (*Myristica fragrans*)

An extract of nutmeg has been proven in at least one study conducted on animals to have the same effect on mating behavior as Viagra does. Nutmeg has been used for a long time in Indian medicine to increase libido. Other spices that are thought to increase sexual desire include cloves, fennel seeds, fenugreek seeds, anise seeds, and black pepper [37].

5.21 Cayenne pepper (*Capsicum annum*), cinnamon (*Cinnamomum zeylanicum*), and ginger (*Zingiber officinale*)

These are aromatic herbs that produce heat within the body and promote circulation in the lower abdominal and pelvic regions. They are used to stimulate one's appetite, both physically and sexually, and are stimulating one's appetite. Vaginal moisture is increased when there is an increase in blood flow to the pelvic region. This leads to an increase in vaginal sensitivity and an intensification of sexual arousal [47, 48].

5.22 Broccoli (*Brassica oleracea*)

Broccoli is an excellent food for increasing a man's libido because it is rich in indole-3-carbinol, a chemical that helps lower estrogen levels (although it can have the opposite effect in women). Additionally, Brussels sprouts are an excellent source of the compound indole-3-carbinol [37, 48].

5.23 Beans (*Phaseolus vulgaris*)

Beans are the best performer when it comes to selecting zinc-rich vegetables. This is true whether the beans are baked, canned, red, lima, kidney, or navy beans. Additionally, they are chock full of protein as well as fiber. After soaking the dry beans, just give them a good rinse to avoid the digestive problems that are often caused by beans.

5.24 Sauerkraut

Isothiocyanates are substances that are produced when cabbage is fermented. These compounds have been demonstrated in tests to inhibit the growth of cancer cells. And if that were not enough, it also helps enhance testosterone production, is loaded with fiber, vitamins, calcium, and minerals, and is packed with all of those things.

5.25 Flaxseeds (*Linum usitatissimum*)

Both flax seed oil and flax seeds themselves have been shown to have several positive effects on sexual health in both men and women. Regular consumption of flax seed helps to enhance testosterone, which in turn leads to an increase in libido and other male sexual traits. Testosterone is a naturally occurring sex hormone that is found in the human body. It is widely believed that flaxseed oil is one of the most effective supplements for enhancing fertility. Because it contains the amino acid L-Arginine, it is an excellent tool for increasing sperm counts. It has been shown that flaxseed oil improves blood flow to the sexual organs, which makes erections last longer [48].

6. Those spices that act as aphrodisiacs

6.1 Cayenne (*Capsicum annum L*)

Cayenne is not just a spice for men's kitchens but can also act as a pain killer and an herb that can warm men up and increase the potency of other herbs. Take cayenne with any of the other herbal aphrodisiacs listed above to help keep blood pressure down and libido up [48].

6.2 Fenugreek (*Trigonella foenumgraecum*)

Fenugreek contains saponins that trigger sex hormones, including testosterone. In a study, 60 men were given fenugreek extract twice a day for 6 weeks, and the libido of these men increased by a quarter. Fenugreek is also used to enlarge the fullness

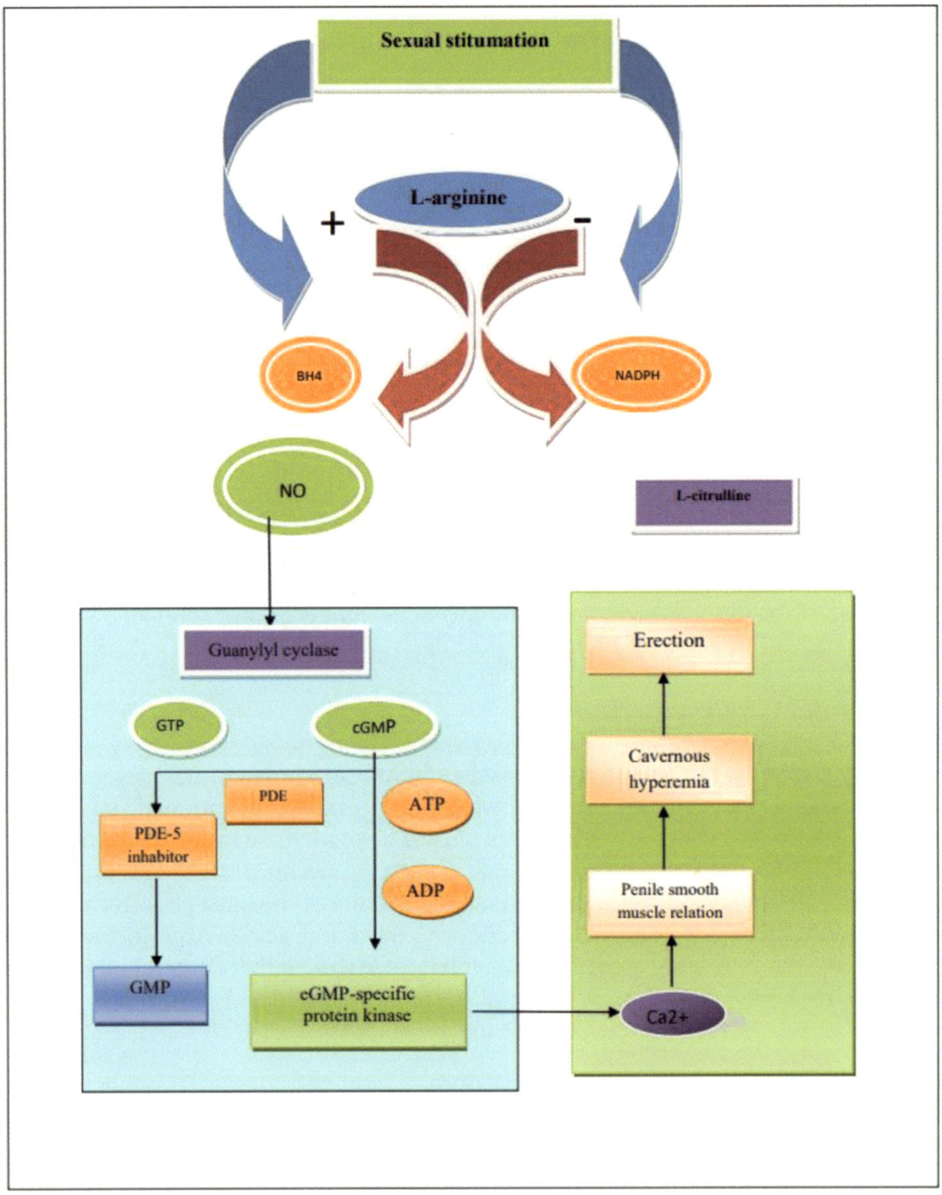

Figure 1.
Mechanism of sexual stimulation [50].

and breast size in women by increasing prolactin. Fenugreek is also used to ease PMS symptoms and menopausal symptoms as well. Also, consuming 500 mg of fenugreek twice a day can help lower blood sugar levels for people with type 2 diabetes. Even though fenugreek is thought to be safe, high doses may cause mild stomach upset [49].

6.3 Garlic (*Allium sativum*)

Garlic improves health and libido drive. Allicin boosts blood flow to men's and women's genital organs. Non-instant. Garlic can improve libido after a month. Garlic increases vigor. It contains heart-healthy vitamins and minerals. Allicin maintains sperm. Raw garlic is preferable, but roasted garlic soup, garlic shrimp, and garlic bread also work. Garlic is libido-boosting. Estrogen-rich foods boost a woman's libido. Estrogen raises sexual desire. Properly dosed garlic supplements may be beneficial [37, 48].

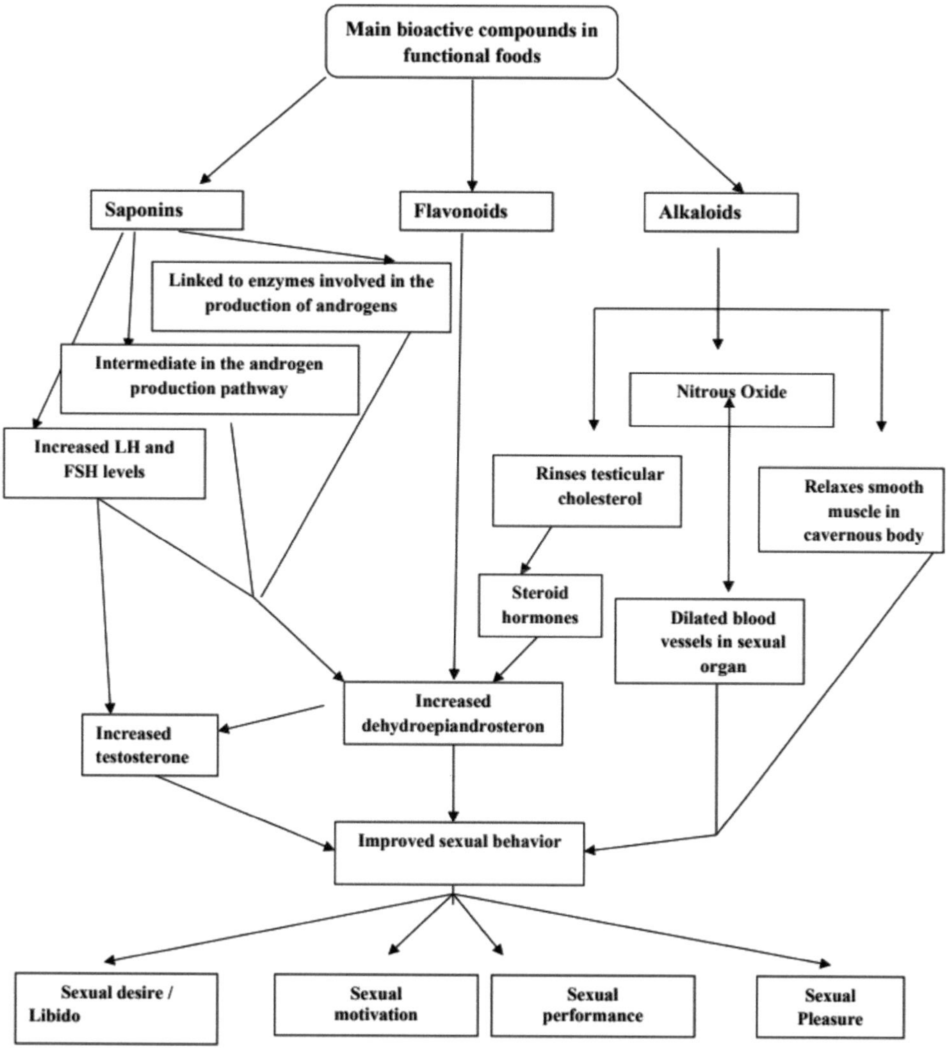

Figure 2.
Functional food stimulation of libido [51].

6.4 Saffron (*Crocus sativus L*)

Saffron is a *C. sativus* flower spice. Traditional benefits include stress relief and libido effects, especially for depressed patients. Studies reveal saffron improves antidepressant-caused sexual dysfunction [48].

6.5 Cardamom

Cardamom has a high concentration of cineole and other antioxidants, both of which improve circulation in the penis and are found in cardamom. This results in an erotic sensation and an enhancement of the overall libido that is sustained for a longer period (**Figures 1** and **2**) [52].

7. Conclusion

Due to alterations in dietary habits and lifestyle factors in the modern period, libido has been shown to significantly decline. To provide the body with vital nutrients, it needs to reclaim its libido. To fully utilize all the nutrients that functional foods provide, it is necessary to make the right selections, put them through the right processes, and use them. To maintain a healthy sexual life, it is necessary to consume foods that are rich in nutrients such as all macronutrients, vitamins A, D, E, C, and B complex, as well as minerals such as magnesium, selenium, zinc, iron, calcium, and manganese, and phytochemicals, herbs, and supplements.

Acknowledgements

We would like to express our gratitude to Ms. Dajana Jusic for her support in the submission of this book chapter. In addition, we would like to thank Ms. Neha Kumari,(BHU)for her comments regarding the drafting of the chapter.

Conflict of interest

The authors declare no conflict of interest.

Author details

Neelesh Kumar Maurya
P.K University, Shivpuri, M.P, India

*Address all correspondence to: neeleshkumar.maurya@gmail.com

References

[1] Oluwole DT, Akhigbe RE, Ajayi AF. Rohypnol-induced sexual dysfunction is via suppression of hypothalamic-pituitary-testicular axis: An experimental study in rats. Andrologia. 2021;**53**(2):e13931

[2] Pfaus JG, Sadiq A, Spana C, Clayton AH. The neurobiology of bremelanotide for the treatment of hypoactive sexual desire disorder in premenopausal women. CNS Spectrums. 2022;**27**(3):281-289

[3] Edinoff AN, Sanders NM, Lewis KB, Apgar TL, Cornett EM, Kaye AM, et al. Bremelanotide for treatment of female hypoactive sexual desire. Neurology International. 2022;**14**(1):75-88

[4] Ibragimov S. The hormone estradiol and what advantages it has over testosterone. In: Collection of Scientific Papers «SCIENTIA». Science of XXI century: Development, main theories and achievements. Helsinki, Finland; 2022. pp. 57-59

[5] Krysiak R, Kowalczyk K, Okopień B. Sexual function and depressive symptoms in men with hypoprolactinaemia secondary to overtreatment of prolactin excess: A pilot study. Endocrinologia, Diabetes y Nutricion. 2022;**69**(4):279-288

[6] Wignall L, Portch E, McCormack M, Owens R, Cascalheira CJ, Attard-Johnson J, et al. Changes in sexual desire and behaviors among UK young adults during social lockdown due to COVID-19. The Journal of Sex Research. 2021;**58**(8):976-985

[7] van Anders SM, Herbenick D, Brotto LA, Harris EA, Chadwick SB. The heteronormativity theory of low sexual desire in women partnered with men. Archives of Sexual Behavior. 2022;**51**(1):391-415

[8] Petric D. The introvert-ambivert-extrovert spectrum. Open Journal of Medical Psychology. 2022;**11**(3):103-111

[9] Muñoz P, Correia S. The great war and the fifth international psychoanalytic congress in budapest: Psychoanalysis in the 1910s. Historia Crítica. 2022;**84**:3-27

[10] Agdari-Moghadam N. A review of the fundamentals. Hoarding Disorder. 2021:**1**(1):29-91

[11] Clephane K, Lorenz TK. Putative mental, physical, and social mechanisms of hormonal influences on postpartum sexuality. Current Sexual Health Reports. 2021:1-3

[12] Gurian M. Lessons of Lifelong Intimacy: Building a Stronger Marriage Without Losing Yourself—The 9 Principles of a Balanced and Happy Relationship. Simon and Schuster; Boy Scouts of America. 2015

[13] Vincent BT, Sztwiertnia M, Koomen R, Warren JG. Discounting for money, food, and sex, over the menstrual cycle. Evolutionary Psychological Science. 2022:1-1

[14] Schleifenbaum L, Stern J, Driebe JC, Wieczorek LL, Gerlach TM, Arslan RC, et al. Men are not aware of and do not respond to their female partner's fertility status: Evidence from a dyadic diary study of 384 couples. Hormones and Behavior. 2022;**143**:105202

[15] Patel A. Sexual health conversations with men. In: Men's Health. Boca Raton: CRC Press; 2021. pp. 174-183

[16] Rudnicka L, Kaczorowska A. Treatment of diseases associated with non-cicatricial alopecia. Dermatology Review/Przegląd Dermatologiczny. 2021;**108**(6):504-516

[17] Montgomery KA. Sexual desire disorders. Psychiatry (Edgmont). 2008;**5**(6):50

[18] Sousa B, Oliveira BM, de Almeida MD. Growth trends in boys and girls (10-17 years old) from autonomous region of Madeira, Portugal between 1996-1998 and 2007-2009. Annals of Human Biology. 2012;**39**(6):526-529

[19] Jaehne EJ, Smith JD, van den Buuse M. Analysis of striatum and brain levels reveals sex differences in conversion of methamphetamine to amphetamine in mice. Neuroscience Letters. 2022:136722

[20] Naji L, Dennis B, Rosic T, Wiercioch W, Paul J, Worster A, et al. Mirtazapine for the treatment of amphetamine and methamphetamine use disorder: A systematic review and meta-analysis. Drug and Alcohol Dependence. 2022:109295

[21] Javaheri A, SaberiZafarghandi MB, Shati M, Roshanpajouh M. Evaluating the effectiveness of short-term clinical guideline to treat sexual addiction disorder in people with sexual addiction: A clinical trial. Iranian Journal of Psychiatry and Clinical Psychology. 2022;**28**(2):1-9

[22] Marcinkowska UM, Shirazi T, Mijas M, Roney JR. Hormonal underpinnings of the variation in sexual desire, arousal and activity throughout the menstrual cycle–A multifaceted approach. The Journal of Sex Research. 2022:1-7

[23] Paulinus CE. A philosophical examination of the concept and nature of infidelity in marriage as a socio-ethical issue in contemporary society. GPH-International Journal of Social Science and Humanities Research. 2022;**5**(07):36-42

[24] Yamuna M, Kumar CS. Bravissimo-M tablets: A scientifically formulated male libido enhancer to restore sexual vitality & to increase spermatogenesis. 2021;**5**(4):23-29

[25] Sim M, Hong S, Jung S, Kim JS, Goo YT, Chun WY, et al. Vitamin C supplementation promotes mental vitality in healthy young adults: results from a cross-sectional analysis and a randomized, double-blind, placebo-controlled trial. European Journal of Nutrition. 2022;**61**(1):447-459

[26] Ali ME, Farag BF, Hussein HA, Fahmy S. Sexual activity, semen characteristics and testosterone levels in mature male rabbits treated with hormonal and non-hormonal preparations. Egyptian Journal of Animal Production. 2022;**59**(2):79-85

[27] Oyareme V, Osaji EI, Bah A. The environmental health benefits of four different selected vegetables (Saluyot Spp, Melissa Spp, Ocimum Spp and Talinum Spp), procured in serrekunda market for cosmopolitan consumption rate in the Gambia. Open Access Library Journal. 2022;**9**:e8974

[28] Dogani M, Askari N, Kalantari-Hesari A, Rahbar FH. The effects of P. atlantica as a libido booster and sexual enhancer on the reproductive system of male rats. Journal of Traditional and Complementary Medicine. 2022;**12**(4):345-353

[29] Stojkovski K, Best HGH. Supplements: Ingredients, benefits, and side effects. Order. 2022;**3**:00

[30] Stewart E. Over the counter and home remedies. In: Sexual Function and Pelvic Floor Dysfunction. Champions: Springer; 2021. pp. 123-136

[31] Nguyen HD, Kim MS. Effects of heavy metal, vitamin, and curry consumption on metabolic syndrome

during menopause: A Korean community-based cross-sectional study. Menopause. 2021;**28**(8):949-959

[32] Ahn TK, Kim JO, An HJ, Park HS, Choi UY, Sohn S, et al. 3'-UTR polymorphisms of vitamin B-related genes are associated with osteoporosis and osteoporotic vertebral compression fractures (OVCFs) in postmenopausal women. Genes. 2020;**11**(6):612

[33] Athira KS, Tripathy TB, Sukumar BS. Ayurvedic food supplements for sexual health: A review article. International Journal of Health Sciences and Research. 2019;**9**(5):347-355

[34] Hamed M, Akhigbe R. P-002 Zinc restores testicular integrity and function in HAART-treated male Wistar rats via modulation of Nrf2/NFkB pathway and downregulation of caspase 3 signaling. Human Reproduction. 2022;**37**(Supplement_1):deac107-deac002

[35] Bindari YR, Shrestha S, Shrestha N, Gaire TN. Effects of nutrition on reproduction-A review. Advances in Applied Science Research. 2013;**4**(1):421-429

[36] Hooshang H, Farahani AV, Rezaeizadeh H, Forouzannia SK, Alaeddini F, Ashraf H, et al. Efficacy of date palm pollen in the male sexual dysfunction after coronary artery bypass graft: A randomized, double-blind, clinical trial. Evidence-Based Complementary and Alternative Medicine. 2022:2022

[37] Zhang D, Jin L, Han J, Song Y, Song H, Lei T. Effect of Bushen Yangluan decoction combined with clomiphene citrate on ovulation and ovarian function in patients with infertility due to polycystic ovary syndrome. International Journal of Clinical and Experimental Medicine. 2021;**14**(2):1095-1102

[38] Wang PH, Li YC, Wu YH, Chen JL, Qiu JT, Yang SH. Clinical evaluation of Guilu Erxian Jiao in treating perimenopausal syndrome. Chinese Medical Journal. 2012;**23**(2):165-181

[39] Danno K, Colas A, Terzan L, Bordet MF. Homeopathic treatment of premenstrual syndrome: A case series. Homeopathy. 2013;**102**(01):59-65

[40] Chedraui P, Hidalgo L, San Miguel G, Morocho N, Ross S. Red clover extract (MF11RCE) supplementation and postmenopausal vaginal and sexual health. International Journal of Gynecology & Obstetrics. 2006;**95**(3):296-297

[41] Khairullah AR, Solikhah TI, Ansori AN, Hidayatullah AR, Hartadi EB, Ram SC, et al. Review on the pharmacological and health aspects of apium graveolens or celery: An update. Systematic Reviews in Pharmacy. 2021;**12**(2):595-601

[42] Purnamasari R, Lusiana N, Widayanti LP, Kumalasari ML. The effectiveness of zinc micronutrients from pumpkin (Cucurbita moschata D) extract on the testosterone levels of mice (Mus musculus L). Indian Journal of Forensic Medicine & Toxicology. 2022;**16**(1):986-993

[43] Olabiyi AA, Ajayi K. Diet, herbs and erectile function: A good friendship! Andrologia. 2022:e14424

[44] Yee A, Uloko M, Goldstein I. Clinical experience with testosterone undecanoate capsules (Jatenzo): The first 50 patients. The Journal of Sexual Medicine. 2022;**19**(5):S128

[45] Varade PR, Jambhale AL, Jadhav AS, Kondilkar MB, Patil KP, Patil BR. Formulation and evaluation of asparagus racemosus granules

for determination of antioxidant activity. 2022;**11**(4):807-814. Available from: https://ndhealth.wordpress.com/2010/12/02/rev-up-your-libido/

[46] IsHak WW, Clevenger S, Pechnick RN, Parisi T. Sex and natural sexual enhancement: Sexual techniques, aphrodisiac foods, and nutraceuticals. The Textbook of Clinical Sexual Medicine. 2017;**1**(1):413-432

[47] Barton DL, Pugh SL, Ganz PA, Plaxe SC, Koontz BF, Carter J, et al. Randomized controlled phase II evaluation of two dose levels of bupropion versus placebo for sexual desire in female cancer survivors: NRG-CC004. Journal of Clinical Oncology. 2022;**40**(4):324-334

[48] Jiang TA. Health benefits of culinary herbs and spices. Journal of AOAC International. 2019;**102**(2):395-411

[49] Koliji T, Keshavarz Z, Zare E, Mojab F, Nasiri M. A systematic review of herbal medicines to improve the sexual function of menopausal women. Journal of Herbmed Pharmacology. 2020;**10**(1):51-60

[50] Chen L, Shi GR, Huang DD, Li Y, Ma CC, Shi M, et al. Male sexual dysfunction: A review of literature on its pathological mechanisms, potential risk factors, and herbal drug intervention. Biomedicine & Pharmacotherapy 2019;**112**:108585

[51] da Cruz AC, Guerra NG, de Souza KEBP, de Castro Eleutério I, da Silva LC, Otoni EG, et al. The action of herbal medicine on the libido: Aspects of nutritional intervention in increasing sexual desire. Nutrire 2017;**42**(1):1-8

[52] Manipriya K, Mallika DB, Dixit AS, Goud UK. Promising herbs as alternatives for women with symptoms of menopause: A review. Journal of Drug Vigilance and Alternative Therapies. 2021;**1**(2):46-64